# Walter Kempner
# and the Rice Diet

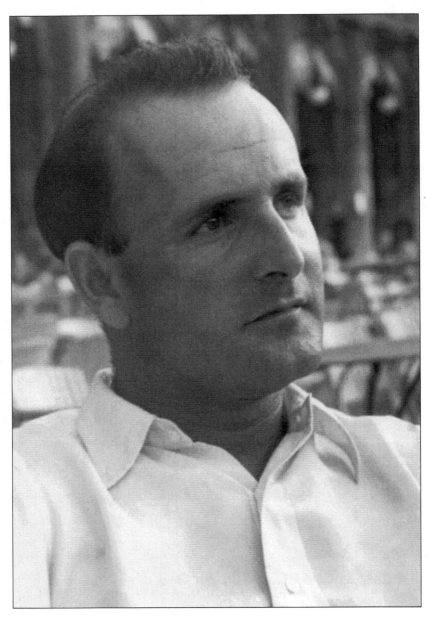

Walter Kempner ca. 1934–35.

# Walter Kempner
# and the Rice Diet

*Challenging Conventional Wisdom*

Barbara Newborg, MD
*with* **Florence Nash**

CAROLINA ACADEMIC PRESS
Durham, North Carolina

Library of Congress Cataloging-in-Publication Data

Newborg, Barbara.
  Walter Kempner and the rice diet : challenging conventional wisdom / Barbara Newborg ; with Florence Nash.
     p. ; cm.
  Includes bibliographical references and index.
  ISBN 978-1-59460-885-8 (alk. paper)
  1. Kempner, Walter, 1903-1997 2. Medical scientists--North Carolina--Biography. 3. Reducing diets. 4. Rice--Therapeutic use. 5. Rice in human nutrition. I. Nash, Florence. II. Title.
  [DNLM: 1. Kempner, Walter. 2. Physicians--Germany--Biography. 3. Physicians--North Carolina--Biography. 4. Diet Therapy--history--Germany. 5. Diet Therapy--history--North Carolina. 6. History, 20th Century--Germany. 7. History, 20th Century--North Carolina. 8. Hypertension--diet therapy--Germany. 9. Hypertension--diet therapy--North Carolina. 10. Kidney Diseases--diet therapy--Germany. 11. Kidney Diseases--diet therapy--North Carolina. WZ 100]
  RM222.2.K4475 2010
  613.2'5092--dc22
  [B]

                                        2010035764

CAROLINA ACADEMIC PRESS
700 Kent Street
Durham, North Carolina 27701
Telephone (919) 489-7486
Fax (919) 493-5668
www.cap-press.com

Printed in the United States of America
2017 Printing

# Contents

# Illustrations

# Preface

In 1939, I was a sophomore at Swarthmore College. My best friend there was Judith Perlzweig from Durham, North Carolina, where her father chaired the Department of Biochemistry at Duke University Medical Center. For spring break that March, Judith invited me to spend some time with her in Durham and meet some of her friends. I accepted with pleasure, grateful to have an alternative to spending all ten days in the rather formal and chilly atmosphere of my own home in New York City. My family was not close.

My train arrived in Durham in the morning, and on that day, as usual, Mrs. Perlzweig had a guest for lunch. Shortly before lunchtime, I remember, Judith and I started walking down the road to meet the guest's car. When it appeared, we ran and jumped onto the running boards to hitch a ride back up to the house. The handsome, beautifully dressed young man at the wheel was Dr. Walter Kempner, brought to the United States from Berlin in 1934 as one of the European scientists and scholars rescued from the looming Nazi threat. A cell physiologist, Dr. Kempner had been offered a research position in the Department of Medicine at Duke's new medical school. The department chairman, Dr. Frederic Hanes, had arranged for him to be housed initially with the Perlzweigs, as Mrs. Perlzweig was German-speaking. Dr. Kempner stayed in their household from October 1934 until May 1935, and he continued to be a nearly daily lunch guest for some years.

After lunch, Dr. Kempner took Judith and me to see his laboratory, and then to a small house where two of his friends from Germany were staying, Miss Fides Ruestow and Mrs. Edit Ullstein Glaser. Over tea and fruit tarts, they engaged in stimulating conversation. Dr. Kempner teased and challenged me: memorize one thousand lines of Shakespeare, identify and locate the major constellations. At some point during my visit, he invited Judith and me to help out in his laboratory, which we did. Our chief task was washing and sorting glassware. I think Dr. Kempner was simply interested to see how we would conduct ourselves in the lab; he was always very curious about people, as I came to learn, and may have wondered whether we had an aptitude for science.

When I got back to Swarthmore after making Dr. Kempner's acquaintance, for the first time in my life I read a Shakespeare play—*Cymbeline*—from beginning to end. Life seemed to be richer than I had imagined. My childhood in New York City had been shaped by a middle-class family that believed mar-

riage to be more or less the only worthwhile aim for a young girl. My parents
had many acquaintances but—so it seemed to me—no close friends, whereas
I had always had a friend or two but rarely any "acquaintances." After my four
days in Durham I felt that new doors had opened, inviting me into new possibilities of friendship and ideas. Many years later, Judith admitted to me that
it had been her hope and expectation that bringing me together with Dr. Kempner and his circle would result in lasting friendships, with just such an effect
on my life.

I was dazzled by these foreigners, by their informed and animated talk.
Dr. Kempner's friends, Miss Ruestow and Mrs. Ullstein Glaser, had fled the
Nazi regime and followed him to North Carolina. On that visit to Durham,
I also was introduced to Dr. Clotilde Schlayer, who had met Walter Kempner in 1920 through his sister Nadja, her friend and schoolmate, and had
come to the United States in 1935 to work with him at Duke. By the time of
my first visit in 1939, a small group of German compatriots and colleagues
in exile had gathered in Durham. After the war, others joined Dr. Kempner
and I became acquainted with them as well. The warmth and closeness of
this group, their wonderful cooking, their sophistication in all things cultural combined with great simplicity of living—all this was powerfully attractive to me. I was spellbound. I started spending parts of my vacations
with the group, working in Dr. Kempner's lab and visiting the circle of émi-
gré friends at their rented summer houses in Kennebunkport, Maine, and
Ocean City, Maryland.

At Swarthmore, I had been pursuing a major in Western European history
with a minor in mathematics, but I had no particular career goals or expectations. My encounter with Dr. Kempner changed all that. Several times he had
mentioned that he thought medicine would be an ideal career for me, and by
my senior year I was convinced. When I told my parents that I wanted to attend medical school, they were less than delighted. Their plans for my future
extended no further than a conventional marriage, though my father might
possibly have envisioned me as a lawyer, his own profession.

I persisted, and after graduating from Swarthmore in 1941, I spent a year
taking premedical courses at New York University. In the late spring of 1942,
I moved to Durham where I found a statistical job at North Carolina State
University in Raleigh and worked part-time in Dr. Kempner's laboratory. I
took additional premed correspondence courses at the University of North
Carolina in Chapel Hill to support my application to Duke Medical School,
which accepted me for entrance in January 1944.

I returned to New York to spend the Christmas holidays with my family before beginning medical school, hoping to achieve some sort of reconciliation

with them over my career choice. While there, I became ill, and it was several months before I was able to return to Durham, by which time I had missed the opportunity to enter Duke Medical School. Instead, I resumed work in Dr. Kempner's laboratory and, with the help of his friends, applied for medical school at the University of North Carolina and was accepted in 1945. After completing my studies at UNC, which at that time offered only a two-year program, I transferred to Johns Hopkins University and received my medical degree there in 1949. Upon graduation I returned to Duke as an intern and then as an assistant resident, and in 1952 I joined Dr. Kempner's clinical staff at Duke.

I worked with Dr. Kempner for forty years, becoming his chief medical associate. My main role was to help him treat patients, but I also struggled to understand his basic scientific ideas, because I saw that his new and—to me—strange concepts represented a revolutionary and eminently successful approach to the treatment of vascular and metabolic diseases. And I, like virtually everyone who encountered him, was fascinated with Walter Kempner himself. He was the most brilliant person I have ever known, broadly educated, charismatic, and unassailably confident. While he was absolutely uncompromising in his fight to reverse diseases long thought to be irreversible, he had great charm and humor and was able to cajole—or, if necessary, browbeat—his patients into following what he himself admitted was an "unpleasant and monotonous" regime, the rice diet. (As he said, "The only excuse for such a therapy is that it works!") He also drew to himself a circle of devoted friends who were themselves extraordinary in many ways. In my long association with him and his companions, I learned first-hand about the politics and culture of prewar Germany, the rise of the Nazis and the diaspora of Jews and other "undesirables," about European history both ancient and modern, and, especially, about the true meaning of friendship and family.

Numerous individuals who played a part in Dr. Kempner's life have been the subjects of research and publication: Eugene A. Stead, Robert Koch, Otto Warburg, not to mention Stefan George, Friedrich Gundolf, and the Stauffenberg brothers. This, by contrast, is the first extensive biographical sketch of Dr. Kempner. During his lifetime the public knew only his medical work and publications; his friendships and his literary and artistic interests remained strictly private. I have undertaken this narrative because I thought it was important to draw together the most important threads of his life as well as his work, and I have been encouraged by close friends who felt similarly. The book is, of course, far from exhaustive, but it may interest future researchers on Dr. Kempner, a remarkable scientist who helped to transform the treatment of cardiovascular, renal and metabolic diseases, and a complex individual through whose life were woven many strands of Western intellectual and political history.

After Dr. Kempner died in 1997, I began to organize and preserve the voluminous documents of his research and treatment of more than 18,000 patients. These records are deposited in the archives of Duke University Medical Center. The entire history of Walter Kempner's rice diet treatment is available there and provides data for historians of medicine. Dr. Kempner published scientific articles from 1927 to 1993; reprints of many of these articles are no longer available. To remedy this situation, they have been collected and republished in a two-volume set [2002, 2004].

The material in the chapters that follow comes from these articles as well as from Dr. Kempner's correspondence and clinical records over seventy-odd years. He was a prolific correspondent, to both friends and patients. Most of the clinical and scientific materials, formerly in my possession, have been deposited in the Duke University Medical Center Archives. Most of Dr. Kempner's personal letters are now in the Württembergische Landesbibliothek in Stuttgart, home of the Stefan George Archive, in the section containing documents of Dr. Clotilde Schlayer and her friends. Dr. Schlayer's letters have been a mine of information as well. My account also relies to a great extent on my own recollection of years of conversations, and stories recounted over the dinner table by Dr. Kempner and his friends. I have verified my recollections where possible with the people mentioned in this book, or with their surviving family and friends, including Judith Perlzweig Binder, Alexander Schlayer, and Katharina Mommsen. I am grateful to Maik Bozza at the Stefan George Archive for his assistance, to Doris Marriott for her tireless and miraculously productive research in the archives, and to Danielle Schmechel, who was a great help in organizing our files for the book. Dr. Frank Neelon gave generously of his time and good counsel, for which he has my warm thanks. In particular, I owe a great debt of gratitude to Joan Mertens, without whom this book would not exist. She too was a friend and admirer of the remarkable people at the center of this story, and she has generously supported its writing with scholarly and meticulous editing. My warmest appreciation goes to Florence Nash who, with endless patience, enthusiasm, sensitivity, and verbal resourcefulness, helped me weave together information from many diverse sources into an integrated narrative.

# Walter Kempner
# and the Rice Diet

# Ricers

In June 1944, at the annual meeting of the American Medical Association in Chicago, a young doctor from a young medical school startled the audience with a report of his highly unorthodox research in the causes and treatment of hypertension and kidney disease. In a poster presentation and address, Dr. Walter Kempner of Duke University meticulously detailed the cases of one hundred fifty patients with acute or chronic primary kidney disease, or with hypertensive vascular disease, whom he had treated at Duke Hospital between 1939 and 1944. He had put these patients—carrying virtual death sentences in an era before the development of drug treatment—on a radically restricted diet consisting chiefly of rice and fruits. For periods ranging from four days to thirty months he followed their progress, scrupulously documenting not only the results of the diet but also his careful monitoring to ensure patients' safety on the radical regime and their strict adherence to it. Over and over, the data showed unprecedented recoveries. Not only was the progression of disease slowed or halted, in many cases the degenerative effects were actually reversed.

Dr. Kempner's claims flew in the face of conventional medical wisdom, and the medical community responded accordingly. They challenged his conclusions, his research methods, even his veracity. Some, unpersuaded even by the abundant charts, x-rays, eyeground photographs, and electrocardiograms that documented his findings, suggested that Dr. Kempner must have somehow falsified them—perhaps switching before-and-after images. But the evidence was clean and indisputable: patients with "incurable" diseases were healing.

Overnight Dr. Kempner and his rice diet became international news. Within the week, inquiries came from the *London Daily Express* and the *Readers Digest*. *Time* Magazine's June 26, 1944, issue included a report on the findings. Articles appeared in the *New York Times*, *Chicago Sun* and *Tribune*, *Miami Herald*, *Detroit Free Press*, *San Francisco Examiner*, *Los Angeles Times*, *Liberty* Magazine, the *American Mercury*, the *American Weekly*, and many others. An Associated Press release on June 12 reported:

**Rice Diet Used to Fight High Blood Pressure. Refugee Places New Drugless Treatment, Backed by Fruits, Vitamin, Before AMA.**

A new entirely drugless treatment for high blood pressure, by a diet of rice and fruit juices, was shown to the American Medical Association today.

The diet is mostly rice, boiled or steamed, plus ample fruit juices and supplemented by vitamins and iron.

Many Duke patients were very ill. Some were blind and had enlarged hearts.

Blood pressures of around 200 dropped immediately on starting the rice diet. Thereafter there was usually a long, slow drop until many patients had pressure within normal ranges and well under 150.

The time of diet varied from weeks to many months, depending on individual reactions. The patients who got better were able to resume limited consumption of meat and eggs but not unrestricted diets.

There were failures and in one group of 127 patients 16 died. But some successes were spectacular. One patient who was sent to the hospital with autopsy papers already signed, recovered. It is the result of four years work at Duke University School of Medicine, and the results in which the majority of cases were helped and many apparently cured were shown in the scientific exhibit by Dr. Walter Kempner, a refugee physician.

The rice-diet treatment is the result of feeding kidney tissues kept alive artificially in glass tubes in the Duke laboratories to test a new theory.

A June 14 release from the Science Services syndicate to over 400 publications in the US and abroad reported:

### Rice Diet Helps Patients with High Blood Pressure and Kidney Disease, Doctors Told

Much attention is being attracted by the report of a diet that seems to help patients with high blood pressure and kidney disease.

Dr. Walter Kempner, of Duke University, developed the diet and reported it to the American Medical Association here. It consists solely of rice, fruit, juices, sugar, vitamins, and iron.

Dr. Kempner's theory is that one of the kidney's functions, that of deaminating the amino acids of protein, is disturbed by lowered oxygen supply and the result is high blood pressure. The rice diet was developed to reduce the amount of protein the kidneys have to handle and thus lower the amount of harmful, abnormal substances which he believes causes the high blood pressure.

Not all patients benefit from the diet, though no ill effects from it have been seen. Blood pressures were reduced in about 60% of the patients, he said. The diet, like that for diabetics, must be prescribed individually for each patient so far as amounts of rice and the other ingredients are concerned....

Patients began flocking to Durham, North Carolina, for the "miracle cure" at Duke Hospital. In time, Dr. Kempner treated patients from Saudi Arabia, Austria, Canada, Belgium, El Salvador, Guatemala, Cuba, Panama, Honduras, Egypt, Cyprus, England, France, Greece, Haiti, Hong Kong, Israel, Iran, Australia, Italy, India, Japan, Jamaica, Bermuda, Lebanon, Mexico, the Netherlands, New Zealand, Peru, the Philippines, Puerto Rico, South Africa, Argentina, Colombia, Chile, Uruguay, Sweden, Spain, Turkey, Germany, Switzerland, and Yugoslavia, and from forty-nine of the United States.

Eventually, the demand far exceeded the supply of beds available to Dr. Kempner at Duke Hospital, so he created external facilities. Two capacious old houses on Durham's tree-lined residential streets were converted to centers where rice patients ate three meals a day and were monitored by Dr. Kempner daily. They also provided bed facilities for patients too ill (or too young; there were many children over the years) to live independently in the community. The other patients, with help from the staff, found their own quarters, many in neighboring boarding houses. The "rice houses" became little communities in themselves, and the "ricers" part of the Durham population. Over time, as a side effect of the rice diet—dramatic weight loss—became increasingly evident, many patients began coming for treatment of obesity. They became a familiar sight in Durham and inspired its nicknames, "Fat City" and "Diet Capital of the World." But the diet's primary work was always the treatment of cardiovascular and kidney disease.

Of more than eighteen thousand patients who came to Dr. Kempner and the rice houses over the years, many are fixed in memory because their stories were moving, or amusing, or amazing. To those of us who treated the patients, the best memories were naturally of those whose response to treatment was most successful. A fifty-year-old movie theater operator from Connecticut, for example, arrived in February 1952 with malignant hypertension: blood pressure 255/141; extensive damage to his heart and eyes; and poor kidney function. He brought a letter from his physician, who estimated his life expectancy at less than one year and suggested that a radical sympathectomy might possibly double that. We started him on the rice diet instead, and after eighteen weeks of following it faithfully, his blood pressure was 178/100, his electrocardiogram (EKG) was—and remained—normal, his eyegrounds were almost normal, and his heart had decreased in size. He returned home to Connecticut but came back to Durham twice a year, for periods of a few days to a few weeks, in which we continued to find him vastly improved except for some evidence of persisting kidney damage.

Fifteen years later, on one of this patient's visits, Dr. Kempner presented him to the Duke Hospital house staff. He introduced him by saying, "Once there were three sick patients who all received a very poor prognosis from their doctor. On receiving the bad news, the first one immediately called his lawyer and accountant to put his affairs in order. The second immediately flew to an expensive resort to lounge on the beach with beautiful young women. The third immediately got another doctor. Ladies and gentlemen, I present that third patient." The patient escaped by nearly eighteen years the death sentence imposed by his own physician.

Another memorable patient—a pleasant fellow full of admiration and gratitude for the rice diet program—turned out to have a more than passing acquaintance with the world of organized crime. One day, in 1948, he happened to hear Dr. Kempner discussing a presentation he was shortly to give before a medical group in New York. Recollecting his reception by the AMA in Chicago four years before, and the ongoing controversy over the rice diet, Dr. Kempner remarked, "I expect there's going to be one tough fight." Taking Dr. Kempner aside, Mr. N. assured him that there would be nothing to worry about: He would be glad to come to New York and bring a couple of his seasoned associates to lend a hand. Dr. Kempner thanked his defender and said that he wasn't worried about physical violence. However, when he stepped up to the podium at the Waldorf-Astoria a few days later, Mr. N., accompanied by several burly men, was seated prominently in the audience, on the alert for action.

A number of celebrities of one kind or another were enrolled in the rice program over the years, and their presence generated stories, some true and some not. Public interest in the rice diet as a successful weight-loss treatment increased sharply when Burl Ives was admitted in late 1963 for treatment of obesity, which he felt was impairing his singing voice. The press followed his progress. Fortunately, he was a conscientious patient and did very well. "I've lost seventy-five pounds in the last four months and I expect to drop another seventy-five pounds by the end of the year," he declared to a reporter for a syndicated article. [Hal Boyle, AP, May 7 1964]

> "I can walk 10 miles a day now and never get tired. Before that I'd puff like a steam engine when I went a hundred yards. I used to have hot pipes"—his term for stomach upsets—"and colds before I went on this diet. Since then I haven't had hot pipes or a cold," Ives said. "I used to have to put down a pound of steak before I went to make a

recording. Now I can eat a few grains of boiled rice and sing like a bird."

In 1968, the wife of the governor of New Jersey, Mrs. Richard Hughes, came to Dr. Kempner for treatment of obesity complicated by diabetes. The October 1968 issue of *The Ladies Home Journal*—at that time a major national publication with high circulation—had blazoned across its cover, "How I Lost 80 Pounds in 19 Weeks, by a Governor's Wife." Mrs. Hughes's long, chatty, and effusive description of her experience on the rice diet pumped up public interest even further.

A persistently repeated tale about the comedian Buddy Hackett is that, in rebellion against the strictures of the salt-free diet, he once broke into the lab and poured salt into the patients' urine samples awaiting analysis. That never happened. I do, however, remember that once, in a hospital waiting room, he commandeered the public address system at the reception desk and called out, "Everyone please lift your legs." The startled patients obediently raised their legs off the floor. Hackett waited; finally he said, "Okay. Everybody put your legs back down." They did. He was a nice man and fond of Dr. Kempner, though he did once refer to him as a "damned Prussian!"

I remember Lorne Greene, who had a short but successful stay with us, saying that the most unpleasant aspect of a career in acting was having to submit to all that makeup every day. A letter he wrote to a colleague describing his rice diet experience is worth quoting as an excellent model for healthy patient attitude toward the program:

.... As for Duke University Medical Centre—yes, I did go there, in 1969. In the 15 days I spent there (it was all the time I had at my disposal) I had a most thorough medical examination, then I went on the Rice Diet at the Kempner Clinic. One is an out-patient. You rent a room in a motel, or hotel, or perhaps you can find someone to share an apartment with. I do not recommend the latter. The more Spartan the existence the better. You go to a place like that to do one thing only: lose weight. And if you do not concentrate on that, then you would be wasting your time and money.

I did not have much time, so I concentrated and did exactly as I was told. I ate only what was put before me. The main course was rice, then a little fruit, and something to drink. In between meals, I'd walk. As much as six hours per day. If someone was around to walk with, fine, otherwise I walked alone, with my little radio playing music or news. In the time I was there, I lost 18 pounds and 5 inches around the waist. Then I took the family to Hawaii and in the next 3 weeks, now eating some chicken and salad and fruit and much walking, I lost another 10 pounds, then I had to film in England, stayed on a restricted diet of salad, rice, fruit, or fish and fruit, and I lost another 12 pounds in 3 weeks. I began to lose so quickly that I put on the brakes, since I didn't want to change my profile during the making of the picture.

The bottom line is, that I found the Kempner Clinic at Duke most effective and it did the job for me.... because I also did the job for it. It's a two-way street. There are no miracles in weight loss. You just have to do it as they prescribe it. If you don't fool around, allow yourself to be induced to go to parties at night, sneak snacks, drinks, sleep late, loll around, then you can make it easily in a month, maybe less. If you are weak-willed and don't do as advised, you'll not gain all the benefit you should from the investment of time and money you are making. What's a month of your life compared to the rest of your life as you would like to see yourself? You may find that they will tell you that you must lose more than 30 pounds. So be it, do it. Work hard and you will succeed and achieve your goal. But you must be most prepared for a semi-monastic life. Oh, you can go to a movie, play bridge, but I know that there are too many people who go there to get away from their misery, and since misery loves company, they find others with the same kind of problems, and they play it up, have the fun they couldn't have at home with the restrictions of living at home. They lose some weight, but not what they should have lost. If your attitude in going there is right, you will be happy for the rest of your life because you will then eke the most out of every moment you are there. I felt marvelous and still do because of my experience there.

When trumpeter Al Hirt was with us, he asked Dr. Kempner if his daughter, one of eight children, could come for treatment as well. Dr. Kempner told him there were no openings, but Hirt was hopeful he might cajole him to change his mind. I remember him walking into a room bearing a huge stack of his recordings, singing "Here Comes the Bribe!" Dr. Kempner's patients included a variety of professional athletes, including the boxer Archie Moore, who was a lovely man. A number of football players and their coaches came to us for pre-season conditioning.

After their stay in Durham under daily supervision, patients were discharged to follow a regime worked out individually for them. Patients whose spouses or staff took the trouble to fix the diet attractively and palatably fared well. Those with families who were either not asked or who were unwilling to support the patient's efforts had a harder time. And reintegration into social lives presented challenges. The temptation to drift gradually away from the strict diet was enormous, especially under the pressure of special occasions: birthdays, weddings, vacations. At times, however, a reminder of what was at stake would come: a rise in blood pressure, a mild stroke, an eyeground bleeding, angina or the illness or death of a friend or relative. Then the patient would get back on track, and the cycle of fluctuating adherence to the rice diet would be resumed.

Usually, patients first returned for check-up after two months, then again after three months, then four, and then five, getting what might be considered a partial and gradual divorce from the program. Eventually most patients reported to the clinic twice a year. On these occasions a complete re-examination was performed: history, physical, blood counts, blood and urine chemistry tests, chest film, EKG, kidney function tests, and, if indicated, eyeground photographs. Depending on the findings, the diet's constraints would then be increased or cut back. While away, the patients were still required to mail in monthly urine samples to Dr. Kempner's laboratory. I found it an impressive testament to the program's renown when I found specimens from Egypt and Cyprus in a single day's mail.

For all of these dangerously ill patients, Dr. Kempner was single-mindedly dedicated to restoring the greatest degree of health possible. Infrequently, patients persistently failed or were unwilling to match his efforts with their own, in which case Dr. Kempner denied them, with the greatest tact, further access to his clinic. But in most cases, Dr. Kempner was able to convince patients that their struggle was indeed one of life and death, and that the regimen, as difficult as it was, would more than repay all the effort.

It is clear that the extraordinary success of the rice diet depended largely on the force of Dr. Kempner's authority—a belief in rigid discipline both for himself and for others. Other doctors who attempted to apply his methods invariably underestimated the technical difficulties and the degree of rigor required; they eventually relaxed their efforts and could not achieve his results. For Dr. Kempner, the ricers would do it. And with his unassailable confidence and will, Dr. Kempner drew to himself a dedicated circle of friends and staff who were almost fanatically committed to his work. Their complete commitment was key to convincing the patients to persevere.

Dr. Kempner's personality brought out in others inner reserves and stamina that they never knew they had. I remember we treated a very well-known Hollywood director, a forceful personality unaccustomed to taking direction from others. He constantly questioned Dr. Kempner's findings and recommendations until, exasperated, Dr. Kempner said to him, "It makes no sense to tell you anything! You are like all my patients from New York and Chicago. If I tell you two plus two equals four, your response will be, 'No, it's three point nine, or four point two!'" A few weeks later, Dr. Kempner overheard a newly arrived patient greeting someone in the next room, "Well! What are you doing here?" He was gratified to recognize the director's voice replying, "I'm here trying to learn that two plus two equals four."

Along with his potentially forbidding intensity, however, Dr. Kempner possessed extraordinary magnetism and charm. As evidenced over and over in his voluminous correspondence, he used humor, personal concern, a gentle insistence on personal responsibility, and a disdain for excuses to persuade his patients to comply with the difficult regimen.

> *To a 54-year-old patient, 1951*: Somebody remarked the other day that everything good and everything bad I get comes from my patients. Looking over the past 5 years I should say that, fortunately, everything connected with you was good. Please take the very best care of yourself so that this will be true for at least the next 51 years.

> *To a 57-year-old patient, 1954*: I hope you are behaving as well as possible and following more the words of wisdom from the mouth of your physician than the desires of your own taste buds. IF YOU COULD BE AS NICE TO YOURSELF AS YOU ARE TO OTHER PEOPLE I WOULD HAVE AN IDEAL PATIENT.

> *To a 30-year-old kidney patient who abandoned the diet when he became a Christian Scientist, 1954:* I can only repeat the advice I gave you: If you want your hands to be clean, you have to wash them, otherwise they will be dirty.... There are things ... that one has to do well, for only if one does them well and gets them out of the way can one be "free" for the higher level. Health is one of these things, like cleanliness, writing addresses right, correctly filling one's fountain pen, and paying one's taxes, and while insufficiency in any of the others may merely be unpleasant, in matters of health it may also be dangerous—and not only for the "lower level" but also apt to extinguish the possibility of giving yourself to those "higher" activities you really want to pursue.

> *1962:* I am afraid that for you there is no easy way to solve the obesity problem. I also do not think your physical and mental health can be definitely improved before you once make up your mind to get out of the driver's seat and let yourself be driven by a competent and reliable man whom you really trust, regardless how rough the road may be and how uncomfortable you might feel during the trip.

*1963*: VERY MANY THANKS for the most beautiful cheesecake with which I celebrated my birthday. (As I told you, you are spoiling your physician too much, but I cannot deny that he enjoys it.) It is really not fair that I am allowed to have these delicacies and at the same time always preach to you that you should almost starve, but I am looking forward to sharing these with you after your disease has completely healed and everything is all right.

*To a patient convicted and sent to prison, 1971*: It is difficult to put our feelings into words at this moment, but from a physician's point of view I must say that I have seen so many tragedies: people who were not able to lift their limbs and had paralyzed bowels or gangrenous legs—I think yours is really not a tragedy but just an unpleasant loss of time. I certainly would rather go through such an assignment than to have a first-rate state funeral as John F. Kennedy had. It will also not be a German concentration camp or an operation for cancer. The main thing: Stay well in every respect and fight it through. Before we turn around very often, you may laugh about it. Be sure to keep me informed about everything. I am 22 years older than you, and you still have at least 44 years to be strong and healthy. With kind regards and best wishes from all your friends here.

Many of his patients, responding to the intensity of his charisma and his caring, became his lifelong devotees and admirers, as their grateful letters attest. Mrs. Jennie Grossinger, the New York philanthropist and hotelier, who was a patient in 1956, wrote:

It is now two weeks since I left Durham, and when I recall how I felt when I first came there compared with my present condition, I … shall be forever and ever grateful to you for it. I also want to say that the loyalty among the members of your staff [was] a great inspiration to me and most helpful. Their devotion and sincerity, in which you set such a wonderful example, is godly. Thank you with all my heart, and again I want to repeat that I will forever and ever be grateful to you.

Patients sometimes responded to Dr. Kempner with what amounted to hero-worship. There was the occasional patient whose devotion was excessive: One wrote (1973), "I've got you sitting right up there next to God." A patient from Egypt wrote (1975), "You have been and will always be for me a spiritual father, a true hope and the helping hand in every single moment when I needed it so much. Thank you for being a great heart and a great physician."

# Family and Early Childhood

Walter Kempner was born on January 25, 1903, in Charlottenburg, a suburb of Berlin. He was the third and last child of Walter Kempner (1864–1920) and Lydia Rabinowitsch Kempner (1871–1935), both eminent researchers in the emerging field of bacteriology. His mother was an especially powerful influence on young Walter. The gifted daughter of a Jewish brewer from Lithuania, she was a forceful, independent personality shaped by her times. She was ten years old when the assassination of Czar Alexander II, in 1881, sparked the most violent anti-Jewish pogrom in Russia in over a century, and it made a lasting impression on her. Her elder son, Robert, recalled that one morning in 1933, he and his mother emerged from their house in Berlin to find the streets transformed overnight by huge swastikas. As they drove to work under the banners hanging everywhere, his mother began to weep with fear. "Now the pogroms will begin here!" *(RMW Kempner 1983, p 135)*

In Lydia Rabinowitsch's youth, higher education was not available to women in either Russia or Germany. She was able, however, to earn a degree in natural sciences from the University of Zurich and subsequently, in July 1894, a doctorate in medical sciences from the University of Bern. In November of that year she joined the laboratory staff of Robert Koch (1843–1910) at the Institut für Infektionskrankheiten in Berlin, a center for the new research on bacterial origins of disease.

After a year with Koch, Rabinowitsch traveled to America in September 1895 to take a course in bacteriology at the Women's Medical College of Pennsylvania in Philadelphia. On December 21, 1895, she was offered the job of setting up and running the college's first bacteriology laboratory. (The laboratory was located within the Department of Pathology since, despite fast-growing interest in the new field of bacteriology, there was still institutional resistance to granting it departmental status.) There, the "brilliant Russian ... with her slight accent and blue-checked bib aprons" became immensely popular with her students, who called her "Dr. Rabby." She twice returned to the Koch Institute, first from August 1 to October 1, 1896, and then again the following summer.

In early 1898, Lydia Rabinowitsch made another advance for women scientists when, in recognition of her being "an especially competent person," the Board of Corporation of the Women's Medical College appointed her Associate Professor of Pathology "in charge of the bacteriological department as Director of Bacteriology, with a seat in the Faculty, at the same salary paid the other professors, $1,150 for the year 1898–1899." Shortly thereafter, she was appointed full Professor of Bacteriology. (*Graffmann-Weschke 1997; Walsh & Poupard 1989*)

Later that spring, the Women's Medical College made Dr. Rabinowitsch its delegate to the International Congress of Hygiene and Demography in Madrid. There she was joined by a colleague from the Koch Institute, Walter Kempner, who had come from Berlin to attend the meeting. Kempner had distinguished himself in Koch's lab by creating, with Professor Ludwig Brieger (1849–1919), the first antitoxin for botulism. It is unclear when the courtship between Kempner and Rabinowitsch began or when these plans were laid, but on April 9, 1898, they were married at the German embassy in Madrid, with no family members present. Then, instead of returning to Philadelphia, Dr. Rabinowitsch, now a German citizen by marriage, resigned from the Women's Medical College and returned with her husband to the Koch Institute in Berlin.

A contentious scientific environment awaited her in Koch's laboratory, now one of Germany's preeminent centers for bacteriological research. In 1882, Koch had postulated that tuberculosis was caused by the tubercule bacillus. This first linking of human disease with a specific organism was not readily accepted by the scientific establishment. Rudolf Virchow (1821–1902), the father of modern pathology and, in the last third of the nineteenth century, one of Europe's most famous physician-scientists, called it "complete nonsense." "People die from tuberculosis because they are weak," he claimed. "A little bacillus doesn't do it." (*RMW Kempner 1983, p 13*) But the bacterial origin of tuberculosis became a prime focus of Koch's investigation. Three strains of the bacillus were identified—human, bovine, and avian; only the human strain, it was generally accepted, caused disease in humans.

Dr. Rabinowitsch had begun investigating the bovine bacillus as early as 1895, before going to the US; her intermittent work for Koch in 1896 and 1897, between visits to the United States, consisted primarily of testing Berlin's milk and butter supply for the bacillus. She entered a three-year contract with the Bolle dairy firm, one of Berlin's largest, to test its products. Tensions arose when, finding tubercle bacilli in some butter, she requested samples of the milk used in its preparation for further testing and discovered that the sample submitted by Bolle had been boiled to destroy any bacteria. She confronted the dairy owner with the doctored evidence, and, according to the story, tapped her forehead as if to say, "Are you crazy? What were you thinking?," whereupon, despite the three-year contract, she was fired on the spot. Her husband took the dairy owner to court on her behalf in a suit that went through three trials before the Kempners finally won the case.

Against expectations, Rabinowitsch had discovered that the bovine bacillus found in milk and butter was identical to the strain present in the intestines of many infants and children who died of tuberculosis. And a test developed by Koch revealed that, in addition to the danger from obviously diseased cows, even milk from tuberculin-positive cows with no evidence of infection could contain virulent, disease-causing bacteria. Rabinowitsch campaigned to have all diseased cows slaughtered and those testing positive for the bacillus, even if disease-free, separated from the breeding herd and eliminated as soon as feasible. All milk was to be pasteurized, in a procedure developed by Rabinowitsch with the Bolle company. The prospect of expensive testing and pasteurization, not to mention the elimination of large numbers of cows, met with widespread resistance in the dairy industry. Moreover, many physicians and scientists still did not accept her findings that bovine bacilli were pathogenic to humans. Even Dr. Koch, who had originally supported his protégé, reversed his stand to side with her challengers at a 1901 tuberculosis conference in London. The controversy, both between science and the dairy industry and internally among researchers, was known as the "Milk Wars," and raged for several years before the unflagging efforts of Rabinowitsch and others finally prevailed, the contaminated cattle were destroyed, and the lives of countless children were saved.

Dr. Koch was away from the Institute from January 1903 until May 1904, pursuing research on sleeping sickness; in October 1904 he resigned his directorship. During his absence, Lydia Rabinowitsch took a two-month maternity leave for the birth of her third child, Walter. When she returned in March 1903, the acting director, Wilhelm Dörnitz, informed her that her colleagues had declared themselves no longer willing to work with her. The reasons are not known. She resigned from the Institute, but retained a loose affiliation that allowed her to follow through with prior commitments, including a series of lectures based on her work there. She then joined Dr. Johannes Orth (1847–1923) in the Pathologisches Institut der Charité, a major research hospital in Berlin, where she remained until 1920. In 1912, the Prussian government appointed her Professor of the Institute of Bacteriological Research in Berlin, the second woman in Prussia to receive a full professorship. In 1913, she became the first woman to edit a medical journal, the *Zeitschrift für Tuberkulose,* a position she held for twenty years, until she was forced to resign following Nazi legislation against Jews. In all, she was author or co-author of more than 60 scientific papers—mostly on tuberculosis—in English and French as well as German. She lectured widely and gave many talks in both Germany and America. In 1920, after her husband's death, she became director of the

Department of Bacteriology at the Moabit Hospital in Berlin, her first paid position, which she held until 1934, when this also was terminated by the anti-Jewish laws.

Dr. Rabinowitsch's accomplishments, remarkable for any woman in that era, were all the more so for a Jewish woman, and her influence extended beyond bacteriology. A staunch supporter of women's rights, she helped set up a fund for interest-free loans to women students. She was a delegate to the Congress of Women in Berlin in 1896 and a speaker before the Women's Welfare Society in 1897. Both she and her husband often traveled abroad to work on public health issues. In 1892 they went to Odessa, where there was an outbreak of plague, and in 1899 to Montenegro to study malaria.

The elder Walter Kempner, Lydia Rabinowitsch's husband, came from a prosperous and cultivated Jewish community in Silesia, in eastern Germany. He graduated from medical school at the University of Munich in 1894 and worked as a volunteer at the Hygiene Institute in Munich and the Senckenberg Institute of the Goethe University in Frankfurt. In May 1896, five months before Rabinowitsch left for Philadelphia, he came to the Institute for Infectious Diseases in Berlin to begin his work with Koch. In time, he became chief physician in the hospital associated with the Institute. It is worth noting that Rabinowitsch and Kempner performed most of their research on a volunteer basis, without compensation, because they were able to live comfortably from his inherited wealth. In keeping with upper-class prejudices of that time, Kempner had exhorted his wife never to work for money, but after his death in 1920 it was necessary for her to accept compensation.

Walter and Lydia Kempner named their first child Robert (1899–1993) in honor of Robert Koch, his godfather, who was a regular visitor in the Kempner home. When I met Robert Kempner in Locarno in the 1980s, he asked me, "What do you think Robert Koch taught me?" Biology, I guessed. Or chemistry? Physics? He smiled and said, "How to fly a kite!" After finishing school in 1917, he entered military service, and late in 1918 he was sent to the western front of World War I. After surviving the terribly high mortality of the war's last months, he took up the study of law at the universities of Freiburg and Berlin and began his legal career in 1923 as a clerk for Erich Frey, a famous Berlin defense counsel. He subsequently spent two years in the public prosecutor's office (1926–1928), after which he joined the Prussian Interior Ministry, where he rose to the position of counsel for the Prussian police. Here he was occupied primarily with the prosecution of politically motivated crimes. From this vantage point, he watched with profound misgivings the emergence of the Nazi party and was openly critical of it, to the point of joining two Ministry colleagues in officially calling for Hitler's deportation in 1930.

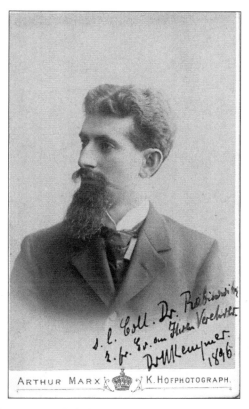

Figure 1. Walter Kempner's father Walter, 1896. Photograph inscribed to his "colleague" Lydia Rabinowitsch "from your admirer."

Less than four weeks after the Nazis came to power, Hermann Goering fired Robert Kempner, on February 24, 1933. From then until 1935, Kempner worked privately as an advisor to endangered persons on matters concerning foreign currency and emigration. On March 12, 1935, he was arrested. The two Gestapo officers who arrived at the Kempner house to take him into custody were courteous; however, the seriousness of his situation was chillingly clear. By good fortune, he was saved from incarceration, or likely much worse, through the indebtedness of a powerful government official, Rudolf Diels (1900–1957). Some years before, Diels, then employed in the "political police" division of the Interior Ministry, had become involved in an altercation with a prostitute, during which he struck her, and then inadvertently left his identification card at her apartment. Diels confessed his situation to Kempner, who predicted that the woman would turn up at the ministry seeking to profit from his embarrassment. Kempner offered to handle the situation and advised Diels to make

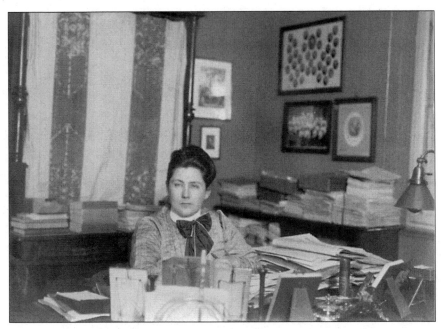

Figure 2. Lydia Rabinowitsch Kempner in her study at home on
the Potsdamerstrasse.

himself scarce. When the woman came, Kempner met with her himself and,
by giving her a sympathetic hearing, persuaded her to relinquish the document. "How much are you asking in damages?" he asked her. "Fifty marks,"
she replied. "Not enough!" Kempner advised her. "You should ask twice that,
and I can make sure that you get it." The woman was delighted. "However,"
Kempner continued, "for that amount you'll have to sign this paper saying that
you will never mention the incident or apply for more payment." The woman
complied, and the grateful Diels expressed his deep indebtedness to Kempner,
declaring that he would welcome any opportunity to repay him.

When the Gestapo appeared at Robert Kempner's door, he knew his best
hope was to get word to Diels, who by then was a Nazi official—a plan he and
his wife had already discussed, anticipating danger to come. Robert asked the
officers if he might shave before leaving, to which they agreed. While he shaved
nonchalantly before the bathroom mirror, he chatted with the waiting officers
as his frightened wife and mother listened from the doorway. As if it were a matter of idle curiosity, he asked them which detention center they were taking
him to, and who was the officer in charge. His wife listened intently to their
responses, and the instant the door closed behind Kempner and the Gestapo

agents, she rushed off to find Diels. He was as good as his word, and Kempner was released—but not before two of his mother's acquaintances had come to console her on the death of her son. They had read in a newspaper that he had been shot. Shortly thereafter, Lydia Kempner suffered a serious, but not fatal, heart attack.

As soon as possible, and without ever returning to the house where he had been arrested, Robert Kempner fled with his family to Italy. They remained in Florence for three years, where he taught in a school for the children of German refugees. Initially, Italy was considered a safe haven for German Jewish refugees. Mussolini certainly did not appear to think much of the Germans. Robert Kempner quoted Mussolini as saying, "We were already a cultured people when they up north were still climbing trees like monkeys." (*RMW Kempner 1983 p 138*) But Hitler's visit to Mussolini in March 1938 changed the situation, and, after Robert Kempner and his wife were arrested by the Italian government and jailed for ten days, they began making arrangements for emigration to the United States. In May 1939, Robert wrote from Italy to his brother Walter, already at Duke University,

> As to staying here, I have at the moment pacified the police with my decision to go to the USA. How long they will be satisfied to wait for that to happen is impossible to say. Any other country—except if necessary England, which is very difficult—is out of the question, since Cuba and the other Central American countries have also closed their borders. We are really not in an enviable position and wait from one mail delivery to the next.

Walter Kempner wrote several letters on his brother's behalf, including one to the Rockefeller Institute. Eventually, the Kempners were allowed to immigrate and they reached the United States in 1939. Robert settled in Lansdowne, Pennsylvania, and became an American citizen. He had a distinguished career as a lawyer, a teacher of European administrative law, and a historian of the Nazi regime. He was advisor to the Roosevelt administration concerning Nazi activities. His knowledge and experience were put to significant use between 1945 and 1949 as a member of the Allied War Crimes Commission and as deputy chief prosecutor of German political leaders at the Nüremberg trials and other war crimes proceedings. Having to spend much of this time in Germany, he acquired an apartment and, eventually, opened a law office in Frankfurt, which became his primary base of operations. His wife, Benedicta, divided her time between Lansdowne and Germany, but until his death, at almost 94, Kempner himself lived primarily in Frankfurt, where he continued to be active in prosecuting former Nazis, including Adolf Eichmann, and in clearing posthumously the name of Marinus van der Lubbe, the young Dutchman who was arrested and executed for having started the Reichstag fire in 1933. Although the Nazis had extracted a confession from van der Lubbe under torture, it is now certain that the blaze had been set by the Nazis themselves. For these activities, Robert Kempner's office in Frankfurt was picketed and his life threatened by neo-Nazis.

Walter and Lydia Kempner's daughter, Nadja (1901–1932), died tragically young of tuberculosis, the very disease her mother worked so hard to eradicate. Though her potential was never fully realized, she too displayed the keen Kempner intelligence and scholarly bent, which she turned to English literature. She completed a PhD at the University of Heidelberg with a dissertation on Sir Walter Raleigh's writings on political theory. She discovered that Raleigh, by incorporating numerous passages from Machiavelli's *Il Principe* and *Discorsi*, had made available in English highly controversial material that was banned in England at that time. (*N Kempner 1928*)

The three Kempner children were nurtured in a rich environment of scientific and scholarly accomplishment. Regular visitors to the household of Walter and Lydia Kempner included not only Robert Koch but other significant scientists as well: Bernard Bang (1848–1932), who isolated the *Bacillus abortus*, and Martin Jacoby (1872–1941), director of the Chemical Institute of Moabit Hospital, among others. Berthold Vallentin (1877–1933), a lawyer, writer, and prominent intellectual, was an uncle by marriage to Lydia's sister Diana Rabinowitsch and close to the family—sometimes entrusted with the care of the young Kempners when their parents were traveling. Vallentin teased the parents for what he considered their excessive anxiety about the children's welfare in their absence. The Kempners recounted the story that, while making their way across Europe by train, they would hear at each stop the telegraph clerk pacing the platform and calling out their name, message in hand. Fearing the worst, they would rush to get the news, only to read, "Children fine. Playing in garden."

As a teenager, Walter Kempner was deeply impressed by the poetry of Stefan George and hoped that he might arrange an introduction through his uncle Vallentin, who was a member of the circle of eminent scholars and artists associated with the charismatic poet. On one occasion, while having tea at his uncle's house, Walter pointed to a photograph of George on Vallentin's desk and said, "Would it be possible for me to meet that man sometime?" Vallentin, aware that the request was impossible, fell silent. He looked around slowly for his monocle. Finally he said to his nephew, "Do have another slice of cake."*

---

* Years later, when Kempner was talking insistently to George and the latter wished for some peace and quiet, he pushed a plate toward Kempner saying, "Do please eat these strawberries." History repeats itself.

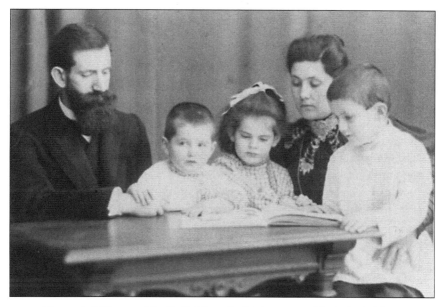

Figure 3. Walter and Lydia Rabinowitsch Kempner with their children
(L–R: Walter, Nadja, and Robert) at home in Berlin ca. 1904.

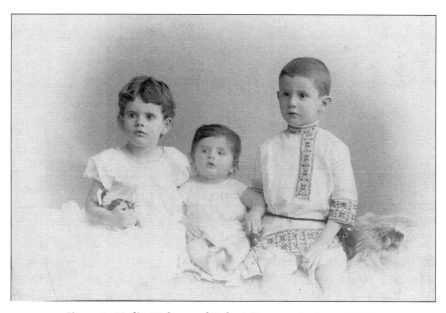

Figure 4. Nadja, Walter, and Robert Kempner in August 1903.

The Kempner household was very practically run. Beggars who came to the door of their house at Potsdamerstrasse 58a in Berlin-Lichterfelde were given a sandwich and a nonalcoholic beverage. This they found unduly parsimonious, and the rumor on the street was that "at the Kempners' 'hunger typhus' is rampant." Their gardener reported to the family that, when he once found a beggar at the door and told him that the family was away, the beggar sniffed, "Gone to Karlsbad on my money!" (Apparently, the notion of entitlement was thriving even then.)

The Kempners, who were not religious, had their children baptized as Christians, a not uncommon practice among Jewish families where societal pressures encouraged assimilation. There are surviving records of Walter's and Nadja's baptism in the Lutheran church; although no evidence is available, it is reasonable to assume that Robert also was baptized. Dr. Kempner told me about receiving religious instruction in school, and recalled that his parents, when the pastor visited the house to discuss their son's approaching confirmation, managed to be absent, leaving detailed discussion of the upcoming event to young Walter and his grandmother.

Kempner's paternal grandmother, Angelika Munk Kempner (1835–1915), lived in the Kempner household and, with both researchers working full time, essentially ran the house. She was a character and, like her grandson, she held firm and precise opinions. A family friend phoned one morning to inquire about his grandmother's health. Walter, who took the call, reported, "Grandmother is quite well today." From another room her strong voice rang out, "How dare you say I'm well!?" Perhaps young Walter learned from her to beware of subjective evaluations.

Walter inherited all of his mother's and grandmother's spirit and more. Bright, curious, independent, he showed his highly individual personality at an early age. He upset his mother by refusing to wear undergarments in cold weather, on the grounds that "Hannibal didn't use them!" He was very fond of lions as a little boy, so he ate raw meat—because, he explained to his mother, it was the diet of lions. She got nowhere by pointing out that he was neither Hannibal nor a lion. One of his mother's many roles was as consultant for a time to the Berlin zoo, which entitled the Kempner children to free passes, and they used them often. Walter's mother gave him a stuffed lion cub from the zoo, which he cherished. Once when Walter was submitting under protest to a haircut, she reassured him that cutting his hair would only make it grow faster. Acting on this new information, Walter shortly thereafter gave his lion a haircut. The shorn lion was relegated to the attic and the disappointed young experimenter learned not to take all statements at face value.

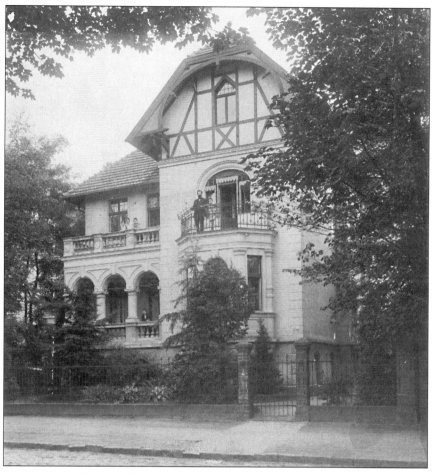

Figure 5. The Kempner house at Potsdamerstrasse 58a.
Lydia is on the left balcony with Nadja and Walter;
Walter senior is at right with Robert; Angelika Monk Kempner is below.

Although Lydia Kempner was an engaged and attentive mother, the constant demands of her research and teaching limited her time at home. She was usually able to return from her laboratory by four o'clock in the afternoon and to spend the rest of the day—except for some editorial work on the *Zeitschrift für Tuberkulose*—with the children. Robert remembered looking at bacteria through her microscope and watching, in their pen under the veranda, the rabbits she used to confirm the tuberculosis diagnosis. The presence of her mother-in-law in addition to household servants helped Lydia maintain a full-time professional career. The circumstances of the children's upbringing fostered their self-reliance and resourcefulness. On one occasion when their mother had to be away for a few days, she left Nadja and Walter money for food. They used the money to buy books instead and ate very sparsely in her absence.

Once, after a swim at a nearby swimming hole, Walter and his brother were lying in the sun, discussing diving, and Robert bet Walter that he wouldn't dive off a high rock nearby. "Of course I would!" said Walter. "Want to bet?" asked his brother. The wager was made. That afternoon, Walter returned alone to the river and, overcoming his fear, dove again and again and again. The next day at the river, Robert reminded his brother of the bet. "What bet?" asked Walter, feigning indifference, and Robert reminded him gleefully, insisting that he follow through or pay up. Whereupon the younger boy climbed to the top of the rock and executed a flawless dive. Later in life he confronted other challenges with the same determination not just to meet but to exceed the challenge.

Walter Kempner had a loving relationship with his father as well as his mother. He remembered that his father, after observing that his son had been unusually still for a long while, asked him, "Are you sad?" The little boy nodded. Without a word, his father took him by the hand, led him to a bedroom, and sat him on his lap. The two sat in complete silence for a while. His father gave him a piece of chocolate; more time passed. Then his father asked, "Are you still sad?" Walter shook his head.

The elder Walter Kempner passed on to his sons an uncompromising sense of justice. His tenacious pursuit of the "Milk Wars" on his wife's behalf was a prime example. Another occurred during a family vacation at Badenweiler, Germany. The spa sponsored a lottery in which, to qualify for the prize, guests had to pledge some amount of money. Kempner senior entered his name and put down five pfennigs. The other guests, unwilling to take this minuscule amount seriously, erased his name from the list, whereupon Dr. Kempner confiscated the entire list and tore it up. The indignant guests took him to court on a charge of "destruction of original documents." He contended to the judge that he had not destroyed an original document; on the contrary, at the instant his name had been crossed off, the document ceased to be the original, and the vandalism in fact originated with the plaintiffs. He won his case.

When Walter was six or seven years old, one of Lydia's brothers visiting the family from Russia took him for a walk in the neighborhood. As they stood admiring the offerings in a candy shop window, his uncle asked him which item he would most want to have. The boy pointed to a huge chocolate June bug— easily over a foot in length—which had been on display in the window for a very long time. His uncle bought it, and Walter brought it home in triumph, to the consternation of his mother. She wiped the dust off and watched anx-

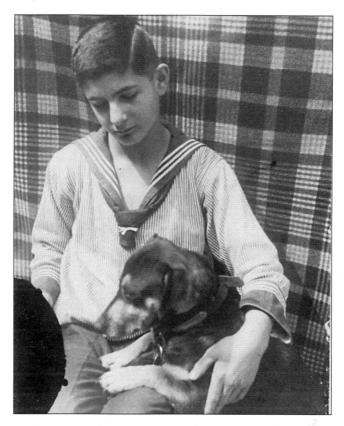

Figure 6. Walter Kempner with his dog Lump, ca. 1911.

iously for signs of distress as the huge confection was gradually consumed. In the early 1960s, reminiscing with a friend, Dr. Kempner recounted the story of the chocolate June bug. From then until his death in 1997, Kempner received in the mail every spring a giant chocolate June bug, filled with pralines, from Hamann, a renowned chocolatier in Berlin.

As a schoolboy at the Schiller-Gymnasium, Walter was repeatedly at the head of his class—the so-called "Primus." He was first not only in lessons but also in instigating pranks. Often he combined the two, as when, chosen to lead the prayers preceding each morning's class, he reduced class time by selecting the longest prayers he could find—which he then recited from memory. When a teacher learned that Walter was tutoring a fellow student, he expressed disapproval at this poor use of his talents and asked, "Couldn't you be spending this time learning something yourself?" Walter thereupon taught himself Norwegian, sufficient to read Ibsen and other authors in the original.

His mother, who professed mock concern that Walter was always at the top of his class, offered him a reward if just for once he would not be first. Finally it happened: although he had again earned the customary "Primus" in his studies, he was demoted to second place because of his mischievous behavior. When he came home and triumphantly claimed his reward, his mother demurred, protesting that a second on those grounds did not count. Her son, however, argued his case, won his point, and was given his reward. His reputation had reached the director of the school, who on one occasion, upon entering Walter's classroom, remarked "*In dieser Klasse ist ein böser Geist, und er heisst Kempner!* [In this class there is an evil spirit, and his name is Kempner!]" An admiring teacher, however, reassured the promising if high-spirited boy that "age doesn't protect from stupidity," and advised his favorite pupil, "Don't keep trying to run your head through a stone wall."

In February 1920, Walter organized an extraordinary tribute for the sixtieth birthday of his favorite teacher, Otto Morgenstern (1860–1942). With a determination and resourcefulness remarkable for his age, he cajoled twenty or so fellow seventeen- and eighteen-year-old students to stage a performance of Sophocles' *Antigone* in Greek, rehearsing secretly and on their own time; he himself both directed and took the role of Kreon. The boys had to learn hundreds of lines in ancient Greek. They borrowed costumes for the production from the Berlin Opera House, with the help of a teacher who had connections there. Attending the performance were students from a neighboring girls' school, including Walter's childhood friend Ruth Lohmann. As the curtain fell and the actors took their bows, she rose from the audience to present young Kempner with a laurel wreath. From a couple of rows behind, she overheard the school director's wife murmur, "Typical Kempner," to which Lohmann loudly retorted, "Thank God!" Walter later turned down a request from the director's wife's for a repeat performance in honor of her husband.

Under the severe privations of World War I, Walter was, like many Germans, malnourished to the point of emaciation. His mother, through her scientific connections, arranged for him to travel in 1918 and several summers thereafter to Tiefhartmannsdorf in south Germany and to Holland and Denmark, where he received proper nourishment.

After her husband's death in March 1920, Lydia Rabinowitsch Kempner took a paid job as director of the Bacteriological Institute of the Moabit Hospital in Berlin. Her elder son Robert was studying law in Freiburg and Berlin; Nadja was studying literature in Heidelberg. Walter, after graduating from the Schiller-Gymnasium in 1920, decided, not surprisingly, to follow his parents' distinguished example and study medicine. In 1921, he entered medical school at the University of Berlin. After only one semester, however, he transferred to the University of Heidelberg, where he received the rest of his medical education, except for two interludes when he went to Berlin for special training, possibly in hematology.

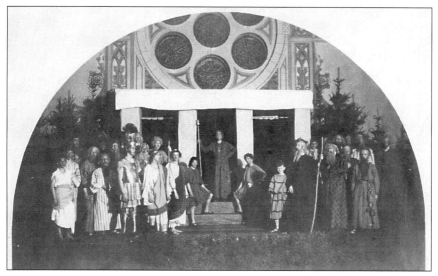

Figure 7. The cast of *Antigone*, the 1920 production by Walter Kempner (center, holding scepter) and his schoolmates at the Schiller-Gymnasium.

# Education: Heidelberg and Berlin

Walter Kempner's medical and scientific education occurred under especially favorable auspices. In the late nineteenth century Germany had eclipsed France and England as the center for science and technology, and, until the rise of Hitler, many of the major advances in physics, biology and chemistry were made there. Two of the most important centers of research were Berlin and Heidelberg.

Kempner's move to Heidelberg in May of 1922 was motivated by his desire to meet Stefan George (1868–1933), a commanding figure in German culture. George was renowned not only as a poet and translator but as the magnetic center of a circle of artists and intellectuals (the *Georgekreis*) united by Socratic ideals of life and art. Shortly after arriving in Heidelberg, Kempner set out to find George. He acquainted himself with George's habits, frequented the places where he usually took his walk, and, one day when George passed by, Kempner ran after him and silently fell into step beside him. George took his arm, and they walked and talked together. After a while, the poet said to him, "And now you will tell your friends you have spoken with me."

"But I have no friends here," Kempner replied. Hearing some discontent in Kempner's voice, George commented, "Some people would be quite happy after such a walk." No, this encounter was simply a matter of luck, Kempner said, somewhat disingenuously, but George replied that the ancient Greeks were wiser: they knew that "*Glück gehört auch zum Charakter*" [Luck is also a part of one's character].* On that day began the most important friendship in Kempner's life, one that lasted until George's death eleven years later. Their contact in these years was intermittent, since George was frequently away from Heidelberg and Kempner was occupied with his medical studies, but it was sufficient for the two men to establish a lasting bond. Their close friendship contributed significantly to Kempner's strong respect for discipline in himself and others, and his reverence for beauty, particularly for the art and literature of Greece.

---

* This story reminds me of a much later one: The cancer researcher Peyton Rous, who developed the mouse sarcoma, visited Dr. Kempner in 1950. As he was leaving, he said to Dr. Kempner, "I wish you luck." Then he turned and reentered the room, correcting himself, "I don't wish you luck. You make your own."

The son of a wine merchant, Stefan George was born in Büdesheim on July 12, 1868, and grew up in Bingen. Extraordinarily intelligent and creative, he was a man born out of his time, and became deeply discontented at an early age with contemporary European society and its modern concepts of progress, technology, and democracy. He found deep resonance in the ideals of classical Greece. The relationship of master and disciple was a key element in George's search for young followers and entailed, at times, homosexual relations.

After graduating from the gymnasium in Darmstadt in 1888, he embarked on extensive travels through England, France, Spain, Italy, Austria, and Switzerland. In Paris, in May 1889, George encountered Stéphane Mallarmé and other French Symbolist poets, who, along with Friedrich Nietzsche, became major influences in his revolt against the realism and romanticism then prevailing in German literature. George believed in art, in its broadest sense, as a means of distancing oneself from the material world, and in the primacy of self-discipline, self-sacrifice, and heroism. He felt that he was a spiritual avatar for his time, one of a succession of divinely inspired voices—Homer, Dante, Shakespeare, for example—who could speak to a new society of intellectual and aesthetic elites. He believed, with Hölderlin, that

> *An das Göttliche glauben*
> *Die allein, die es selber sind.*
> [Only those who are divine believe in the Divine. Hölderlin: *Menschenbeifall*, p 90]

From one of George's own poems,

> *Breit in der stille den Geist ... dass ...*
> *Du nicht mehr still bist und taub*
> *Wenn sich der gott in dir regt.*
> [In the stillness spread your Spirit so that you no longer are silent and deaf when the god in you stirs. From *Der Stern des Bundes*, p 370]

George never had a home of his own, preferring to travel about Germany and Switzerland as a house guest of his growing circle of friends and admirers. In the early years, he went often to Paris and Brussels, as well as various places in Holland, and Italy. Initially he received support from his family; later, royalties and the hospitality of friends enabled him to live an independent, unpretentious, non-bourgeois life. He avoided all publicity, and his early books were privately financed. As a vehicle for his own writing and that of friends and contemporaries whom he respected and wished to encourage, George established a literary review, *Blätter für die Kunst* (1892–1919), through whose pages George and his chosen collaborators gradually became known.

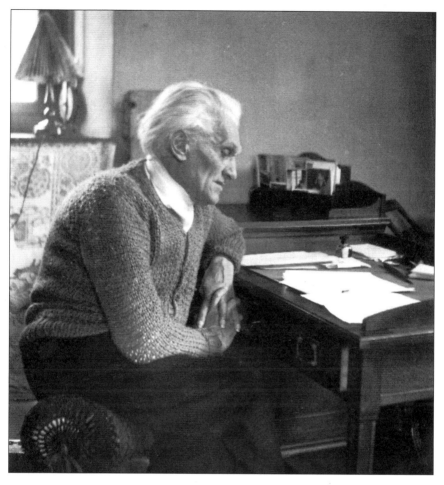

Figure 8. Stefan George.

The writers, artists, and musicians who became part of the *Georgekreis* constituted a remarkable following. His most steadfast, long-lived partisan was the writer and critic Karl Wolfskehl (1878–1948). Perhaps his most gifted disciple was Friedrich Gundolf (1880–1931), whom Wolfskehl introduced to him in the spring of 1899. Gundolf was a literary historian, best known for works on Goethe, Julius Caesar, George, and Shakespeare. He and George produced a new translation of Shakespeare, departing from the classic version by Ludwig Tieck and Friedrich Schlegel. For about twenty years George and Gundolf had a complex and intense relationship, based on profound mutual respect

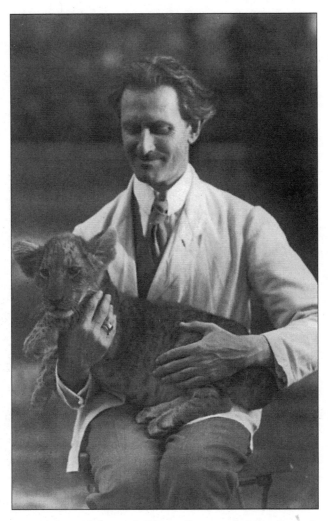

Figure 9.  Friedrich Gundolf in Berlin, 1927, holding lion cub.

and affection but not without tension. George broke off their friendship when Gundolf decided to marry.

Gundolf became a close and influential friend of Walter Kempner, who, despite the rift between Gundolf and George, maintained a close bond with both men until their deaths. (Kempner took it as a good omen that he, Gundolf, and George had all been born on a Sunday.) When Kempner came to Heidelberg in 1922, he was galvanized by Gundolf's lectures; later he described how he perched on the edge of his seat fairly bursting with excitement. Whenever possible, he traveled with Gundolf to hear him speak, and to participate in his search for rare books.* Kempner said that, on one of their early trips together, Gundolf was carrying two fairly large pieces of luggage as they walked to the train station. Kempner took one of them and staggered under its weight: it was full of books. When they stopped briefly to look at something, Kempner willingly relinquished the suitcase and made no protest when Gundolf strode off again with both of them, apparently oblivious to the burden.

Other young people in Heidelberg's university community were fascinated by Gundolf's erudition and personality. Some of Kempner's closest friendships were formed in this group, which included his sister Nadja and her friend Clotilde Schlayer as well as Gerda von Puttkamer (later Schlayer's sister-in-law) and Barbara Zielke (later the wife of Hans Stefan Schultz). They attended lectures and some classes together and met for meals at the university dining hall. When Friedrich Gundolf ate with them, after studying the menu he would invariably order "*das letzte Halb*," a half-portion of the last, and least expensive, item on the menu. Clotilde Schlayer and Nadja did not necessarily follow his example; they ate heartily and often stopped at one of the pastry shops, where they indulged their taste for sweets and carried something away to be shared with the others.

Gundolf had an exceptionally playful, humorous temperament, which manifested itself in short impromptu poems, dashed off in minutes and often accompanied by drawings. He addressed many of them to Kempner—and Kempner's Great Dane, Magog—as well as to Clotilde Schlayer, Nadja, and Barbara Zielke, a testament to their friendship and his skill in light verse. Gundolf's landlady in Heidelberg, comparing Gundolf and Kempner, said, "The professor, he is a good person. He sees how one really is. But the doctor, he's a devil." Gundolf's death on July 12, 1931—George's sixty-third birthday—was announced in one newspaper with an editorial posing the question, What was the greater ill, the death of Friedrich Gundolf or the recent economic crisis? Kempner, devastated, took the news of Gundolf's death to George in Königstein, and remarked, "One should not love anyone too much." George answered, "You might as well say one should not breathe."

Friedrich Gundolf's younger brother, Ernst (1881–1945), an artist, was also a member of George's circle and a friend of Dr. Kempner and Dr. Schlayer.

---

* After Gundolf's early death in 1931 Dr. Kempner acquired some of his considerable library. In 1983 he bought at auction Gundolf's collection of works by and about Julius Caesar. He later offered this collection to the University of Heidelberg, which was unable to accept the gift. In 1996 Dr. Kempner donated the Caesar books to the Duke University Library. After Dr. Kempner's death much of the Gundolf collection, including manuscripts of Gundolf's own works, went to the Stefan George Archive in Stuttgart.

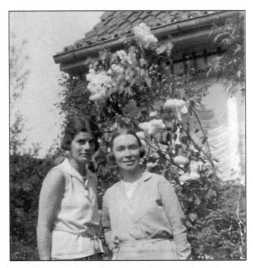

Figure 10. Nadja Kempner and Clotilde Schlayer at the
Boetticherstrasse house, ca. 1930.

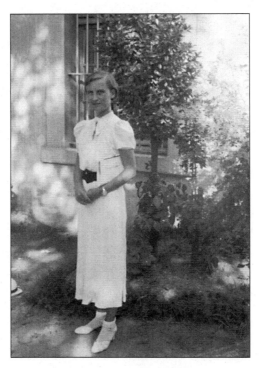

Figure 11. Barbara Zielke (later Schultz).

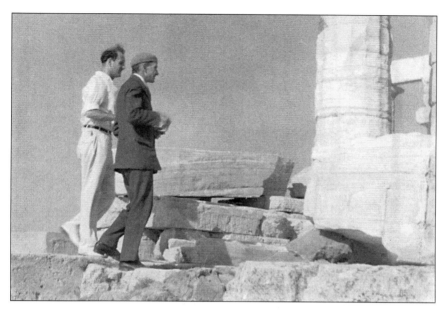

Figure 12. Ernst Gundolf and Walter Kempner in Greece, ca. 1932.

He served as a critical reader for many publications by George's friends. He was drawn to Chinese painting and the work of Aubrey Beardsley, and for years he produced every morning a small landscape, usually a black-and-white drawing. Unlike his brother, Ernst was quiet and withdrawn. He suffered from tuberculosis and went annually to a sanitorium near Davos for treatment, while continuing to live in his parents' house in Darmstadt. Whenever he came to Berlin, particularly after 1931, Ernst visited Clotilde Schlayer at her house in the Boetticherstrasse, which had been purchased for her by her father. Once the Nazis came to power, his appearance there could have created some risk for Schlayer, as the Gundolfs were Jewish. Reluctant to leave Germany despite the danger, Gundolf was for a time imprisoned in the Nazi concentration camp at Buchenwald, but his aunt Gertrud was able to negotiate his release. Once freed, he presented a friend, Edith Landmann, with two of his drawings and asked, "Do you see any difference?" When she found none, Ernst pointed out that one was made before his internment and the other after he got out. In other words, he had been able to maintain himself intact through that experience. He emigrated to England in 1939 and died there in 1945 following an automobile accident.

Clotilde Schlayer (1900–2004) became a life-long and intimate friend of Walter Kempner's. By coincidence, many years before she became a school-

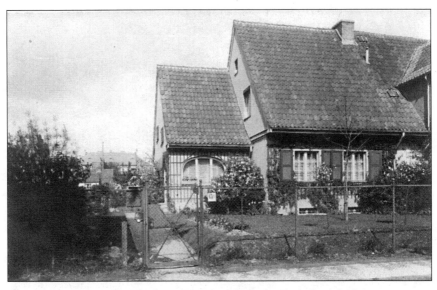

Figure 13. The house at Boetticherstrasse 15c, bought by
Felix Schlayer for his daughter Clotilde.

mate of Nadja's, through whom she met Kempner in 1920, she and her twin
brother Karl, on family vacation at Badenweiler, had come across a park bench
with the inscription "*Für Dr. Lydia K.*" Dr. Schlayer recounted later that she
had been intrigued to find that a woman was so distinguished as to have her
own park bench. The inscription, indeed, referred to Kempner's mother. The
Schlayer and Kempner families both vacationed at Badenweiler, though not at
the same time, and they were not acquainted. Once introduced, Clotilde and
Walter quickly became close, and they often walked and talked together. Not
until three years into their acquaintance did either one of them mention George,
whereupon each disclosed that his writings were an integral but private part of
their lives. From then on, and especially in the early thirties, this shared interest
played a great role in their friendship.

Starting probably in 1922, and continuing for many years, they traveled together in Germany, during university breaks and summer vacations. Years later,
in the 1970s, I believe, Dr. Schlayer gave Dr. Kempner, as a birthday gift, a
collection of postcards documenting their visits to Bamberg, Nürnberg, Weimar,
Dornburg, Loreley, Naumburg, Ulm, Augsburg, Regensburg, München, Wim-
phen, Lauffen am Necker, Heilbronn, Maulbronn, Esslingen, Stuttgart, Worms,
Mainz, Bingen, Bacharach, Oberwesel, Limburg an der Lahn, Trier, Hildesheim,
Halberstadt, Goslar, and Quedlinburg. During 1928 and 1929, they made two

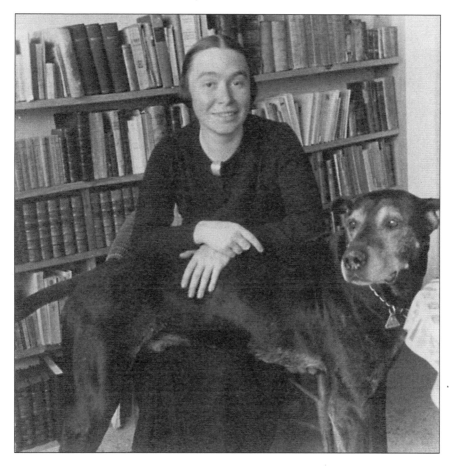

Figure 14. Clotilde Schlayer with Magog in the house
on Boetticherstrasse, Dahlem, 1930–31.

trips to Greece. On their return from one trip they were delayed in Italy because
Kempner had contracted dengue fever. On another occasion they telegraphed
Kempner's mother, "*Leben teuer* [Life expensive]!" In light of Greece's unsta-
ble political situation at that time, Lydia Kempner found this message alarm-
ing, imagining even that it was perhaps a signal that they were being held for
ransom. It was, however, merely an announcement that they needed more
cash, which they duly received. During the twenties, they traveled to visit the
Schlayer family in Spain.

On one occasion in Germany, when young Clotilde was out walking with
her uncle Carl and her father, the uncle made a comment to which she took

exception. She offered her own view, whereupon he said, "To have such a point of view, you must be either very rich or very intelligent." She retorted, "Fortunately, I am both!," a remark that delighted her father. As the conversation continued, her uncle said, "You shouldn't say anything against the Conservative Party until you know something about it." "But I do know about it," his niece retorted, and proceeded to rattle off the details of recent scandals.

Clotilde Schlayer spent 1926–27 in Würzburg, supposedly working on her doctoral dissertation in Spanish literature, but chiefly procrastinating. Coming by to visit and check up on her progress, Kempner found her surrounded by magazines. To motivate her to write, he began to drop by more frequently, always demanding that she read to him what she had written since his last visit. Schlayer completed her work and received her PhD at the University of Heidelberg in 1928, with a dissertation on "Traces of Lucan in Spanish Poetry." (*C Schlayer 1928*) Her later literary publications consisted of Spanish translations of sixty of Stefan George's poems in a bilingual edition (*C Schlayer 1964*) and in 1981 a book of her own poetry. (*C Schlayer 1981*)

Her father, Felix Schlayer (1873–1950), was a businessman and self-taught engineer who lived in Spain from 1895 until his death, with interruptions for World War I and the Spanish Revolution. His memoir, *Ein Schwabe in Spanien*, was edited by his grandson, Alexander Schlayer, and published posthumously in 2007. (*F Schlayer 2007*) He is credited with bringing Spain's agrarian economy into the twentieth century by introducing modern agricultural machinery. On moving to Barcelona, Schlayer was hired by a dealer in farm machinery related to the wine industry; he became junior partner in 1897 and expanded the business to general agriculture. In 1902, when the firm moved from Barcelona to Madrid, Schlayer was invited by King Alfonso XIII to give a private demonstration of the machines for the royal family. According to Clotilde Schlayer, her father found the young king to be both enterprising and interested.

The business thrived; machines were imported from England, Germany, and America. Between 1898 and 1913, Felix Schlayer traveled extensively throughout rural Spain demonstrating the use of harvesters, threshers, and other farm machinery, often modifying and repairing them himself. With hotels or inns rarely available, he shared crowded sleeping benches, feet-to-head, in primitive surroundings. He bought out his partner in 1910 and became sole proprietor of the business. When World War I broke out, the English firm with which he dealt, Ruston Proctor & Co. of Lincoln, severed their connection, and he was forced to deal with German manufacturers (Krupp, Lanz, and Hanomag) in order to maintain the needed supply of equipment for Spain. In 1931, he tried to sell his idea for a new thresher to International Harvester in the United States. His contact was a Mr. Messenger, whose son appeared years later as a patient at the Rice House, where he and Dr. Schlayer were delighted to discover their fathers' connection. Felix Schlayer traveled to America to negotiate the transaction, but again the times were not favorable, and the deal fell through. In 1935 his firm failed.

In 1907, Schlayer had been asked to assist in building a new school in Madrid, partly for German students. He was interested chiefly because of his twin children, Karl and Clotilde, who until then had been tutored at home. The school was built and opened in the fall of 1909. Clotilde Schlayer remembered her first day there, when the girls and boys were assigned to separate classrooms. The students were asked to state whether their religion was Catholic or Lutheran. She had no idea, but noting that most of the other German girls claimed Lutheranism, she did so as well, then waited with trepidation to learn Karl's choice. To her relief, he had also placed himself in the Lutheran group.

Notwithstanding his German birth, in 1910 Felix Schlayer was appointed Norwegian Vice Consul and commercial attaché to Spain. When he protested that he knew no Norwegian and had no idea what to do, he was assured that the office was chiefly honorary and he would only have to sign an occasional paper. At the onset of the Spanish Civil War in 1936, from the dual vantage of his diplomatic position and his wide-ranging travels, he became uneasily aware of mounting evidence that the Spanish government was murdering political prisoners, including some of his friends. Searching for evidence, he repeatedly visited prisons in Madrid and actually discovered mass graves in the countryside, where he saw human limbs sticking out of dirt-filled drainage ditches. He put himself in ever greater jeopardy with persistent challenges to police and government officials—who dismissed him with smiling reassurances—and repeated attempts to alert international humanitarian groups. Spurred in part by Schlayer's efforts, the diplomatic corps in Madrid issued a collective protest to the ruling junta, but the only response was an ominous statement in the Madrid press that all such rumors were "lies and calumny" and anyone guilty of spreading them risked the death penalty.

Finally the pressure on Schlayer became too great, and in 1936 he realized that he urgently needed to leave Spain. As the government began calling for his arrest, he made his way with his wife to Valencia, whence he had booked passage to Marseilles. Just as he drove up to board the boat, the arresting officers arrived in pursuit. However, because he was in an automobile with Norwegian diplomatic plates, he was technically in Norwegian territory, and his pursuers could not touch him. Despite their insistence he refused to leave the car, and thus by this hair's-breadth maneuver escaped to France and ultimately to Germany. There, in 1937–1938, he wrote an account, *Diplomat im Roten*

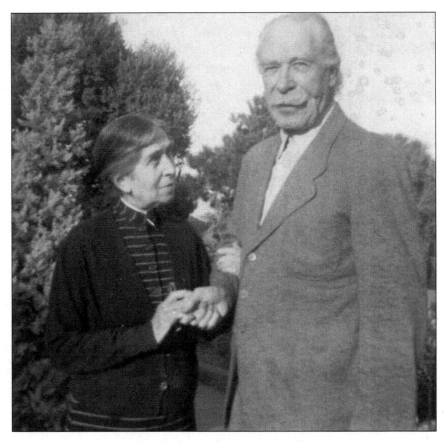

Figure 15. Felix Schlayer and his wife, Rosa Albagés y Gallego,
in their garden at Torrelodones, Spain, ca. 1950.

*Madrid* [Diplomat in Red Madrid] (*F Schlayer 1938*), which was a condem-
nation of the Spanish war crimes. Schlayer was able to put his diplomatic connections to good use in helping both Jews and non-Jews emigrate from Germany.

Felix Schlayer's wife was a singer from Seville, Rosa Albagés y Gallego
(1867–1961), who gave up her career when their twins were born. Concerning her rather individualistic children, she once exclaimed "*Ich bin ein Huhn
das hat gehabt Gänsen!* [I am a hen that has given birth to goslings!]" On her
ninetieth birthday, her son gave her a rocking chair. Astonished, she asked,
"You mean for me to sit here at the window like an old woman?!" Shortly thereafter she tried to give the gold cross she always wore to Rafaela, the housekeeper from Avila who had been with her for many years. "Oh, no, madame!
The longer you wear it the more it will mean to me."

Walter Kempner and his fellow student Gerda von Puttkamer (1901–1953) met in Heidelberg when they arrived simultaneously at a birthday celebration for Friedrich Gundolf. While waiting for someone to answer the doorbell, the two chatted briefly, then Kempner suddenly rushed off and left her waiting on the doorstep. Misinterpreting Kempner's abrupt abandonment of her—to buy Gundolf some last-minute flowers—Gerda (nicknamed "Puma") had sharp words for him when they met the next day in the university dining hall. Despite this inauspicious beginning, they became life-long friends. As a daughter of landed gentry in Pomerania, Puma was expected to lead a conventional existence of marriage and motherhood. Her life, however, followed a different path, in part because of the influence of her elder sister, Annemarie von Puttkamer, who had broken away from the family to become a writer and translator (specializing in American literature) in Munich.

Puma convinced her parents to let her study in Berlin, but when rampant inflation hit Germany, her family instructed her to return to Pomerania at once, as they could no longer send her money: it lost substantial value just in the time it took to arrive. But Puma stayed put, tutoring Russian immigrants in German to cover her expenses. Her students paid her in rubles—one per lesson— which she immediately converted to Reichmarks and spent, knowing that they would be devalued if she waited even a few hours. Sometime in the early 1920s, she met Friedrich Gundolf and another member of George's circle (probably Ernst Kantorowicz, or possibly Arthur Salz or Karl Wolfskehl) while visiting a spa with her mother. The two men persuaded her to come to Heidelberg to study, where she majored in medieval history and became an expert on medieval Sicily. She wrote her dissertation, in 1927, on Pope Innocent IV. Kempner told us that one day, when she complained to him of a headache or cold, he had said, "I hate sick people." "Then," she retorted, "you are eminently suited to be a physician."

Unable to leave Germany and realizing that she would fare better under the Nazis if she had a profession, Puma enrolled in medical school at Freiburg in 1932 and graduated on September 1, 1939, the day the Germans bombed Warsaw and World War II burst upon the world. She never completed the thesis for her medical degree but, in the exigencies of war, she received clearance to practice medicine—first at the regional hospital in Stolp, then in a private women's clinic in Freiburg, and finally in the Department of Pediatrics at Freiburg University. She married Clotilde Schlayer's twin brother Karl in 1927; their son, Alexander, was born March 23rd, 1929, in Freiburg, and since 1962 has lived in Sweden, where he taught school for many years. After the war, Puma and Dr. Kempner resumed correspondence. On her last trip to Europe, in 1992, Dr. Schlayer arranged for Dr. Kempner and Alexander to meet in Locarno, their first contact

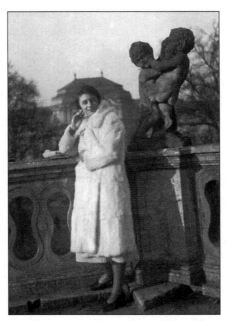

**Figure 16. Gerda von Puttkamer.**

since Alexander was a child of four. Afterward, the two men saw each other several times in Durham when Alexander came to visit his aunt Clotilde.

Through Puma, Kempner met Barbara and Christa Zielke in the early '20s. They were the daughters of the mayor of Stolp, a county seat of some 35,000 inhabitants about six miles from the village where the Puttkamers had their estate. Both were close friends of Puma; in fact, they acquired the nicknames "Nebenpum" and "Orepum," respectively, or "Near Puma" and "Little Puma." In 1923 Christa (1904–1968) married Horst von Roebel (1896–1964), who eventually became director of Rob Forberg, a venerable music publishing house in Leipzig owned by his uncle. As specialists in ballet music, the Forberg publishers had early connections with Tchaikovsky's Russian publishers and later acquired rights to works of Stravinsky, including *The Firebird*, and to Rimsky-Korsakov's *Le Coq d'Or*.

Trained as a gynecological surgeon, Christa von Roebel visited the United States twice before 1939. She had arranged to start working with Dr. George Whipple, dean of the medical school in Rochester, New York, but the war intervened and she was trapped in Germany. Despite her anti-Nazi convictions, she survived the regime without grave danger because she was Aryan and because she successfully avoided anything political. After the war she obtained a position as acting director of obstetrics and gynecology at the University of

Leipzig, in the Russian occupied zone. By means of a perilous trip through the salt mines under the city, she was able to make her way into the American sector of Germany and from there finally to leave for Durham in 1949.

Not all her experiences were grim. In the summer of 1937, Dr. Kempner took Christa von Roebel to the horse races in Torquay. (He had emigrated to the United States by this time but was traveling in Europe on his summer vacation.) Kempner surveyed the list of horses running and, solely on the strength of the name, decided to place a bet on "Briefcase." Dr. von Roebel remonstrated, "Won't you even look at the horses?" The answer was no. When the race got under way, Kempner urged Briefcase on, calling his name loudly, while his neighbors scoffed at his optimism. But—of course—Briefcase won. The only other time that Kempner gambled, to my knowledge, was in 1984, mid-Atlantic on the Queen Elizabeth, in the aftermath of a violent storm. While Dr. Schlayer collected storm pictures from the photographer, Dr. Kempner stopped in at the ship's casino to try his luck with three quarters she had given him. No sooner had he inserted the first coin and pulled the lever than there was "a most satisfactory metallic sound" as twenty dollars in quarters poured forth. The question as to which of them should claim the jackpot was not quickly settled.

In 1931 Christa's sister Barbara Zielke Schultz (1901–1988) obtained her PhD at Heidelberg with a dissertation on the emerging role of Turkey in the European political community. While in Heidelberg, she too became a friend of Friedrich Gundolf, at whose birthday party in June 1926 she and Clotilde Schlayer first met, beginning a friendship that lasted until Barbara's death sixty-two years later. She was able to leave Germany before the war by taking a position in Istanbul as tutor to the family of Arthur Salz, a political scientist and endangered anti-Nazi who was a good friend of Friedrich Gundolf.

While pursuing his medical studies in Heidelberg during the early twenties, Kempner lived in various places, including a narrow, three-storey house quite near the castle. He told us that when he took his first lodgings as a medical student, his landlady announced that she expected to die soon. Her mother and her grandmother had each died at age 50, she explained, and she was 49. Kempner offered her a prescription: walk up a nearby hill every day and sit there for an hour before returning. She did as he said and, with the benefits of regular exercise, a period of peaceful reflection, and, no doubt, the effect of his very confident instruction, she lived on.

At the completion of their studies, the medical students were divided into groups of four for the qualifying examinations. Each group met with the examining professors on a rotating schedule. Dr. Kempner particularly remembered one of his partners, a student named Zernick, because of his performance in an oral pharmacology exam. When the professor asked Zernick to discuss the classification of laxatives, the young man froze; finally he blurted out, "Peppermint water?" "That may be a favorite household remedy in your family," the professor said dryly, "but it is not considered a significant laxative."

In the 1960s when Clotilde Schlayer and I were traveling together visiting sites of Romanesque architecture in France, we found ourselves in Sarlat, a village in the Dordogne. She spotted a pastry shop across the street and went to investigate the baked goods in the shop window. After studying the pastries she looked at the adjacent door plate and noticed the name Zernick. On an impulse, we rang the bell. Indeed, this turned out to be the very same Zernick, Dr. Kempner's old exam partner.

Dr. Kempner told us that when he and his fellow students were discussing with another professor the schedule for their dermatology examination, the professor suggested a time, and Kempner pointed out that they had already scheduled a different examination for the same hour, with Professor G. The other students gaped at him in horror: Professor G. had died over a year earlier! How could Kempner have been ignorant of this? In the German university system, once students had registered and paid their fees, it was not obligatory for them to attend classes if they preferred to study on their own, and Walter Kempner had, typically, taken full advantage of this freedom. One would think, however, that he might at least have ascertained whether the professor was alive or dead.

One of the requirements for the doctoral degree in Germany was a research paper. Kempner chose to study the effects of fasting and of various chemicals, including insulin and adrenalin, on the blood sugar levels of laboratory animals with induced diabetes. (*W Kempner 1927a*) Insulin, a substance normally produced by the pancreas but which also can be synthesized in the laboratory, helps regulate blood sugar. Too much insulin can dangerously lower blood sugar levels and even lead to convulsions. Kempner found that, in his experimental animals, he could produce very low blood sugar through fasting, in the absence of insulin and without causing convulsions. Relevant to the future development of the rice diet, he also found he could raise blood sugar levels with injections of adrenalin. Because the adrenal gland responds to sodium, its activity is decreased by removal of sodium. These observations on adrenalin later bore fruit when they helped lead Dr. Kempner to the idea that sodium might play a role in both diabetes and hypertension via the adrenal glands and, more important, that maximal restriction of sodium could contribute to the treatment of these and other diseases.

When he showed his dissertation to his advisor, Dr. Ludolf Krehl (1861–1937), the latter commented, "It's very interesting. Now write the paper." Dr. Krehl was responding to the fact that the document consisted almost entirely of graphs, tables and charts. It was Dr. Kempner's style, then and thereafter, to handle data in the most concise, efficient possible way. He added two or three sentences only to the paper, which then was accepted. Later at Duke, he confounded his colleagues with his famous "yellow charts," medical records that consisted of daily recordings of patients' lab findings to the virtual exclusion of any written comment.

In 1926–27, following completion of his studies, Walter Kempner served his internship under Dr. Krehl, who directed the medical clinic at Heidelberg from 1906 to 1933. Looking back on his time with Krehl, Dr. Kempner told us that his own name apparently had been incorrectly listed in enrollment records, so that for a time Krehl addressed him as "Herr Kestner," an error he did not bother to correct. Krehl seemed to take satisfaction, Kempner said, in having discovered real medical talent in an obscure young man. When Krehl finally learned his intern's real name and realized who his parents were, he exclaimed, "*Kempner war doch verlogen!* [Kempner was a damned liar!]"

Krehl was not only an outstanding physician but also one of the earliest promoters of the integration of natural sciences with medical research. Krehl also oversaw the founding of the Kaiser Wilhelm Institute for Medical Research in Heidelberg, one of several government-supported institutes dedicated to scientific research in various fields. At the time of its founding, the Rockefeller Institute in New York was the only other research center focused on applying research in the natural sciences to medical practice. Krehl began recruiting key scientists in 1927, but their work was confined to his laboratories at the university of Heidelberg until the new building opened in 1930, with Krehl as its director.

During his internship, Kempner was offered a position on the medical staff at the Rockefeller Institute in New York. Krehl may have encouraged the offer, because Kempner had shown considerable aptitude for the integration of natural science with medicine, and because of his mother's reputation as a prominent researcher. When the offer came, Krehl said to Kempner, "*Wenn Sie diese Stellung nicht annehmen, werde ich Sie mit allen Tiernamen nennen!* [If you don't accept this position, I will call you every kind of animal!]" Despite the threat, Kempner did not accept, principally because he did not want to move so far away from Stefan George, who by this time was consulting him about his medical needs. Upon completing his internship, in March 1927, Kempner went instead to Berlin to interview for a position as research associate to Otto Warburg (1883–1970), director of the Institute for Cellular Physiology in Berlin-Dahlem.

Dr. Kempner told an amusing story of how he came to join Otto Warburg. He had been working late one night in Krehl's laboratory when he fell into conversation with the janitor, a Mr. Ziegler, who was none too impressed with the industriousness of the Heidelberg medical faculty. "Here in Heidelberg, everybody wants to be Professor and wants to teach and wants to talk," the man complained. "There never was anybody here who wanted to work. When something finally has to be done, they shout, 'Herr Ziegler, Herr Ziegler!' Doctor, I get sick to my stomach when I hear my name." Amused, Kempner queried him further, and the janitor allowed that in fact there had been one hard worker, a fellow named Warburg, but he had left Heidelberg and not been heard of since. Kempner looked up some of Warburg's papers in the library and was intrigued. Discovering that Warburg was working at the Kaiser Wilhelm Institute of Cellular Physiology in Berlin, he decided to go to see him and ask for a position.

During the interview Professor Warburg asked him, "Do you know any chemistry?" No, Kempner replied. Any physics? Again no. But, Kempner added, he had written a paper on phlorhizin diabetes. Warburg considered, and said, "We have no room here, but you can sit in a corner and observe for two weeks." At the end of that time, Warburg asked Kempner, "Have you now learned our methods?" No, Kempner replied. "How long do you think you would need to stay here in order to learn them?" Two years, said Kempner. Warburg assented, and Kempner spent the next year and a half, until October 1928, working in Warburg's institute.

Otto Warburg, known as the father of cellular physiology, received the Nobel Prize in Physiology in 1931. Through the techniques and apparatus developed in his laboratories, it became possible to study the function of living cells, that is, the actual physical and chemical reactions associated with cell metabolism and how these reactions affect cell life. Prior to Warburg, cell function had been identified only in terms of changes in appearance, composition, and migration. Warburg pointed out that the essential sources of energy for human body cells lie in two chemical reactions—respiration (oxygen consumption) and fermentation (the splitting of sugar into lactic acid). Investigating the nature of the enzymes involved in these processes, Warburg found that, whereas normal cells cannot live without oxygen, cancer cells thrive in its absence, deriving most of their energy from glycolysis, that is, fermentation.

Presumably at Dr. Warburg's suggestion, Dr. Kempner began his work at the Institute on the respiration of plasma in chickens infected with plague virus, apparently his first time focusing on respiration. He published his finding that plasma in normal chickens shows no respiration, but plasma of plague-infected chickens does. He concluded that this respiration was either of the virus itself or induced by the virus. (*W Kempner 1927b*) At the end of this paper, Dr. Kempner wrote, "For advice and help, especially with regard to the bacteriological investigations, special thanks should go to Frau Professor Rabinowitsch-Kempner."

Otto Warburg and Walter Kempner were well matched, both in the focus of their scientific interests and in their forthright empiricism. Years later, in a tribute to his mentor, Kempner wrote, "Great scientists can be very average and boring people. Warburg was interesting."

> In 1927, my first year with [Warburg], I discussed in the evening with Dr. Krebs the results of an experiment I had just made that day. "There must be a mistake," Krebs said. I questioned why and he answered, "This is against all the laws of cellular physiology." The next morning when Warburg had come in, he asked me for the results of my experiment. I showed it to him and he said in English, "That's very exciting." I argued, with my newly acquired wisdom, "But it can't be true; this is against all the laws of cellular physiology." Warburg pondered a moment and then said, "Of course you have to repeat it six or seven times, but if it always comes out the same, the laws of cellular physiology have to be changed." (*W Kempner 1984 p26*)

Dr. Kempner repeated the experiment, obtained the same results, and the laws were duly changed. This was a significant breakthrough for a young scientist. Unfortunately, there is no evidence in the records of which experiment this was, or which laws it overturned.

When Dr. Kempner joined Warburg's institute, he probably first stayed with his mother at the family home in Lichterfelde, a Berlin suburb. In late 1927, Clotilde Schlayer, who lived in Berlin on and off, invited Kempner to use her house at Boetticherstrasse 15c as his residence. Stefan George, on his frequent sojourns in Berlin, also began staying at the Boetticherstrasse house as Dr. Kempner's guest. George and Schlayer did not actually meet, however, until February 1931, when she was invited to read from her Spanish translations of George's works at the Achilleion. This was the atelier of the art historian and sculptor Ludwig Thormaehlen (1889–1956), which functioned as a meeting and working place for the George circle in Berlin. When after a time George interrupted her reading, Schlayer protested that the best translations were yet to come. George, greatly amused by this, nonetheless declared the session over for the day. A few days later, a promising young friend of his, Johann Anton (1900–1931), committed suicide, and George absented himself from the group for a while. Schlayer did not see George again for some months, nor did she return to the Achilleion.

She bought a car—a 1928 Oakland—so that Kempner could drive George to the gatherings at the Achilleion and elsewhere. To break in the car and accustom himself to it, Kempner made a trial run on a winding, hilly road. He found the steering quite strenuous and later discovered that he had had a flat tire. When

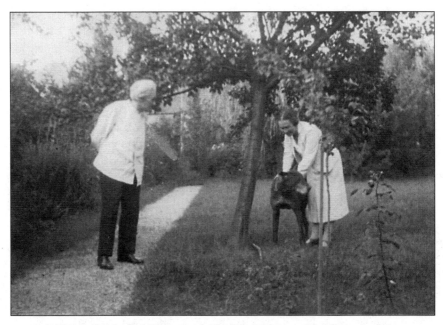

Figure 17. Stefan George and Clotilde Schlayer with Magog in the
garden at Boetticherstrasse, ca. 1931–32.

it was fixed, driving became easier. Later, he told us that, on the night after that
first drive, he dreamt of fighting the steering wheel to keep the car on the road.

For Kempner and his friends, auto trips were often filled by recitations of
poetry, a predilection that began with George. Once while driving George,
Kempner launched into a long declamation, perhaps from Schiller's *Don Car-*
*los.* George asked, "Tell me, were you once an actor?"

While he was working at the Warburg Institute, Kempner became acquainted
with Dr. Hans Gaffron, an associate there. Gaffron approached Dr. Kempner
one day to ask if he would please examine a mysterious swelling on his sister
Mercedes's neck. Kempner looked at the swelling and decided it was nothing
more than an irritation from her violin. As playing was more a diversion than
a serious pursuit, she decided it was simplest to give up the instrument. This
initial encounter resulted in a long association between Mercedes Gaffron and
Walter Kempner. As she lived in a suburb near Dahlem, they saw each other
frequently. Through her he met Fides Ruestow, then a student of photography, who also became a friend and associate.

Dr. Kempner left the Warburg Institute in 1928 under circumstances that are
not entirely clear, but apparently had to do with a conflict over Warburg's want-

ing Dr. Kempner to present his results at a meeting. Dr. Kempner refused, but Dr. Warburg entered his name on the program anyway and may have presented Dr. Kempner's findings himself. Dr. Kempner left the institute shortly afterward and spent the next five years, from November 1928 to April 1933, as an assistant to Gustav von Bergmann (1878–1955) at the Charité Hospital in Berlin, as both physician and scientist. Bergmann, who like Krehl was a leading clinician, was struck with young Dr. Kempner's skill in treating patients and soon promoted him over more senior colleagues to a paid position* as assistant physician. Dr. Kempner not only saw patients but also was put in charge of one of the wards. He continued the work on cell physiology that he had begun under Otto Warburg.

Kempner was joined in this work by Ernst Peschel and Ruth Lohmann (his admirer at the school production of Sophocles' *Antigone*), both still medical students. Together they wrote three papers on inflammation: metabolism and inflammation (*Kempner & Peschel 1930*), cancer metabolism and inflammation (*Lohmann 1931*), and the biology of inflammation (*Lohmann 1938*). All of these relied on Warburg's apparatus and methods to examine the chemical reactions of living cells. In order to investigate experimentally the specific reactions of inflammation, Dr. Kempner created a model environment by producing blisters on the skins of both healthy patients and those with a variety of illnesses. The blisters were induced by applying canthariden, a strong irritant, to the skin. The blister sites responded to the irritation with an influx of white blood cells, or inflammatory cells, to the site. The life and death of these cells produced in the site a fluid characterized by a number of changes, including decreased concentrations of oxygen and sugar, and increased acidity. Dr. Kempner assumed that the blister would exchange fluid with normal tissue surrounding the site, maintaining equilibrium, but the blister was a walled-off system, and there was little or no exchange. This study of the chemical changes in inflammation, summarized in the following paragraph, was perhaps the most significant of the early investigations undertaken by Dr. Kempner and his associates.

---

* After this promotion, he called his mother and asked, "If something happened, would it change anything between us?" His mother assured him that nothing could disturb their relationship. The following week, when Kempner came to take his customary Sunday lunch with his mother, she contained her curiosity until the end of the meal. As she was going to her desk to write her weekly check for Kempner, he proudly told her that he had a paying job. She turned and said, "Then you won't be needing this any more." "But Mother," Kempner reminded her, "You promised that nothing between us would change." "Ah," she exclaimed. "Now I see!" And the weekly allowance continued.

The formation of acid and decrease in energy-supplying substances bring about the death of inflammatory cells and destruction of tissue (necrosis) ... These reactions are destructive not only to the inflammatory cells but also—when the inflammation is not, as in this experiment, sterile—to the bacteria that brought about the inflammation.... Thus, in some illnesses, inflammation can have a predominantly healing effect through the destruction of bacteria; in others, inflammation inflicts harm through the destruction of body tissue. One should therefore consider both the healing and harmful effects of inflammation on the entire organism and try to increase or decrease the inflammatory reaction according to whether the greater danger comes from tissue destruction or from bacterial spread. (*Kempner & Peschel 1930 p 454–455*)

Dr. Kempner found that, in diabetics with an elevated blood sugar concentration, the sugar in the blister fluid decreased—just as it does in nondiabetics—but still remained high. The persistent high concentration of sugar might explain diabetics' decreased resistance to infection.

With Dr. Kempner's guidance, Ruth Lohmann wrote a paper on cancer metabolism and inflammation (probably the dissertation for her MD degree). She postulated that, since tumor cells rely on either respiration or glycolysis (fermentation) to grow and since, as Dr. Kempner observed, inflammation reduces both these energy sources, then inflammation should inhibit the life and growth of tumor cells. She placed rat sarcoma cells in inflammatory fluid, with minimal oxygen, for periods of six and ten hours, then placed the same cells in rat serum with normal oxygen concentration. The metabolism in the cells exposed for six hours was greatly reduced; in cells kept ten hours without oxygen, it was practically zero. This means, she wrote, that

the tumor tissue had died within ten hours under conditions of inflammation, while the tumor tissue kept in serum under constant conditions still exhibited its original metabolism.... Ideally, for prevention and treatment of tumors, one should maintain the inflammatory propensity of the body so that degenerating cells, as they appear, will be destroyed by isolation, starvation, and acidity. One should also fight the degenerated cells by increasing the inflammatory capacity. (*R Lohmann 1931 p 7*)

However, Dr. Lohmann cautioned against any "premature illusions of therapeutic realization" in treating cancer by inducing inflammation. In this connection, I was fascinated as a young physician by a patient who had both lung cancer and a lung infection (empyema): when the infection was active, the cancer went into remission.

At Dr. Kempner's suggestion, Dr. Ernst Peschel studied leukemic cells in preparation for his doctoral dissertation. He found that, in contrast to cancer cells and damaged white blood cells, leukemic cells derived their energy from oxydative respirations, and glycolysis does not take place if oxygen is present. (*Peschel 1930*)

For his work on inflammation, Dr. von Bergmann singled Kempner out in his book on functional pathology:

> In my clinic, Kempner studied the metabolism of inflammation in its physical chemical reactions, using and modifying the exact methods of Otto Warburg; as material he used cantharidin blisters, which were familiar to him from Kauffmann's experiments. The presentation of the course of inflammation reminds us of the epoch-making discovery of Pasteur on fermentation of yeast, in which alcohol is produced from sugar. (*Bergmann 1932 p 171*)

These early observations of changes in oxygen, sugar, lactic acid and bicarbonate concentration led to studies of their effects on other cells, including bacteria, plant and organ cells. It was the reaction of kidney cells to low oxygen tension that led eventually to the development of the rice diet.

At the Charité Hospital was a young social worker named Edit Ullstein (1905–1964), whose family owned the powerful Ullstein publishing house. Noticing the attractive young doctor, she introduced herself to him and invited him out to her house with his friends. Kempner reputedly said to her, "I only accept invitations to houses with tennis courts." Not a problem, she replied; she had a tennis court. He, along with Ruth Lohmann and Ernst Peschel, became frequent visitors to Edit's house. Ruth was said to be a very good tennis player.

When neither George nor Gundolf was in Berlin, leaving Dr. Kempner more time for visiting, he saw Mercedes Gaffron and Fides Ruestow from time to time. It was probably in 1928 that he sent the two of them to the Boetticher strasse house to meet Clotilde Schlayer, whom they did not yet know. Fides Ruestow told me, in 2002, that he instructed them to sing this little ditty to Dr. Schlayer on their arrival:

*Was müssen das für Bäume sein wo die grossen*
*Elefanten spazieren gehen ohne sich zu stossen!*
[What kind of trees must those be where large
elephants stroll underneath without bumping themselves!]

Barbara and Christa Zielke occasionally came to Berlin. After Nadja Kempner contracted tuberculosis, she stayed at times in a sanitorium, but when she was in Berlin she made her headquarters in the Potsdamerstrasse house with her mother and visited at Boetticherstrasse. Gerda von Puttkamer Schlayer, on at least one occasion, came from Wasserburg with her two children to visit the Boetticherstrasse. The advent of George's sixty-fifth birthday, in 1933, gave rise to one episode in which Christa Zielke played a leading role. The new Nazi regime had expressed its intention to celebrate the poet's birthday with an official party, but George, anxious to fend off any association with the Nazis, asked Kempner to organize instead an intimate dinner at the Boetticherstrasse house. George's proposal gave him little notice, so Kempner was concerned: the housekeeper was away, Clotilde Schlayer was away. Who would prepare the dinner? He phoned Christa Zielke in Leipzig, whom he knew to be an excellent cook, and asked if she could provide a roast and trimmings. He also asked her to disguise herself as a maid when she came, because George and his closest circle were accustomed to dine alone. Christa complied, and arrived at the house to prepare and serve the birthday meal successfully transformed into a serving-girl—except that she drew the line at replacing her silk stockings with coarser cotton ones.

In April 1933, when the first anti-Jewish laws were enacted, Professor von Bergmann was pressured to fire all the Jewish physicians on his staff. He offered Dr. Kempner a chance to stay, but Dr. Kempner refused the offer. Instead, after a few weeks' vacation, he returned in May to the laboratory of Otto Warburg, with whom he had by this time settled his disagreements. There he took up the study of enzymatic butyric acid fermentation. (*W Kempner 1933a, 1933b*) He remained at the Institute until December of that year. Through letters, Dr. Kempner stayed in touch with his mentors, Bergmann and Warburg, for many years, although, after his emigration to America in 1934, he returned to Germany only once, in 1935, to see his mother; she died that August.

In 1942–43, the Charité Hospital in Berlin was virtually destroyed by bombs, and Bergmann moved to Munich in 1945 to head the Department of Medicine in the university hospital (here, he taught Dr. Kempner's friend Hanna Ruestow). Bergmann continued to follow with great interest Kempner's achievements in cellular physiology and with the rice diet. For a publication celebrating Bergmann's seventy-fifth birthday in 1953, Dr. Kempner contributed an article on the rice diet. (*W Kempner 1954b*) The two men continued to follow each other's work and to correspond. Some of their letters are in Duke's History of Medicine Library, others in the Württembergische Landesbibliothek in Stuttgart.

In 1983, Germany issued a commemorative stamp in honor of the centennial of Otto Warburg's birth. For the occasion Dr. Kempner contributed to the North Carolina Medical Journal an essay remembering his years with Warburg:

In 1968, the year he became 85 years old, he sent me a letter for my 65th birthday and wrote, "In many respects I found that age is better than youth. The fight for existence is over, and, if one possesses luck and reason, one can still live for many years. A bank account is desirable, a house of one's own is desirable, the possibility to do scientific work is desirable. I assume that you have all of this in ample measure. And so I dare to congratulate you."

"Luck and reason." But I think I would never have been lucky in any endeavor in medicine without those years, 1927, 1928, and 1933, with Otto Warburg. (*W Kempner 1984 p 26*)

# Crisis and Diaspora

One afternoon in mid-September 1931, Dr. Kempner and Stefan George were walking in the neighborhood of the Boetticherstrasse. Not for the first time, George expressed his displeasure with Berlin's "*triste paysage*," the relentless gray skies hovering over the city—both literally and figuratively. Well, replied Dr. Kempner, why doesn't *der Meister* simply go somewhere else where it is nicer? The Riviera, for example. After some consideration, George pointed out that there were also quite nice places in the south of Switzerland—Locarno, for example. Kempner reported this exchange to Clotilde Schlayer and asked her to find a place for George in Locarno. Although she had actually met the great poet only once, when she read at the Achilleion, she was, like Kempner, a devoted admirer and committed to serving his interests. The very next evening she took the train to Locarno, where within two or three days she found a promising house, the "Molino del Orso," located in the nearby community of Minusio. She telegraphed Dr. Kempner: "If a rushing brook would not bother you, a charming house." On September 19, she signed a lease, and on returning to Berlin she concocted, with Kempner, an enthusiastic letter describing her find, ostensibly written by her to him from Locarno. Kempner took the letter to George, who was pleased by her description of the house:

> The house sits in a large garden on a steep slope by a rushing stream. It has three levels, each with its own entrance. The highest level would make a suitable apartment, with two comfortable rooms, the larger of which has a balcony overlooking the Lago Maggiore and mountains. The dining room is on the middle floor, the kitchen below.

Remaining in Berlin only long enough to gather the items necessary for setting up a new household, Schlayer returned to Locarno with her housekeeper, Frieda Reichmann, to help with the preparations. Although the lease bore Clotilde Schlayer's name and was financed partially by her money (which was still arriving steadily from her father's business enterprises in Spain), George contributed substantially to the upkeep of the house. On October 1, 1931, Dr. Kempner escorted George by train to Locarno and remained a few days before returning to Berlin. Kempner had expected that George, as was usual for him, would stay for two to three weeks; in fact, he was there for seven months, until

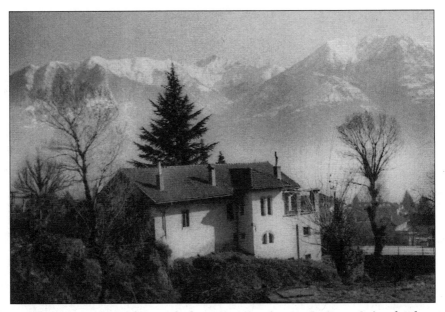

**Figure 18. Molino del Orso, the house in Minusio, near Locarno, Switzerland.**

May 1, 1932. George returned to Locarno on November 2, 1932, and stayed again until March 12, 1933. He made his last visit on September 30 of that year, and never left. On November 26 he had a stroke and on the following day was admitted to the hospital in Locarno, where he died on December 4.

Assisted by the invaluable Frieda, Clotilde Schlayer ran the household during all of George's sojourns, except for a few short absences to visit her parents in nearby Merano. When Dr. Kempner visited, for several weeks at a time, he occupied the smaller room in the apartment. Schlayer had a small alcove off the dining room, and Frieda slept downstairs near the kitchen.

A few days after George's arrival in October 1931, Victor Frank (1909–1943), George's companion during this time, arrived, and he remained part of the household during most of George's stays. Dr. Schlayer's almost daily letters to Walter Kempner describe the routine at the Molino house. George ate breakfast in his apartment with Frank, after which the two men took a walk, weather permitting. He then read a number of newspapers, including the *ABC,* a prominent Spanish paper, and dealt with correspondence. George appeared for lunch in the dining room promptly at noon. The menus for the midday and evening meals were planned and written out by Schlayer and prepared by Frieda. During mealtimes the conversation was lively. In the afternoons George was again with Frank, sometimes with other guests as well, and often he took a second walk. George was a connoisseur of tobacco and wine, and after the noon and evening meals, he and Frank rolled cigarettes for themselves. Twice a week and on special occasions George gave Schlayer a "*verdienst*" cigarette, or "cigarette of merit."* After dinner, he reclined on the sofa and discoursed, with prolonged pauses, on a wide range of subjects. Schlayer said she had the impression that he was speaking from a great distance. After a month or so of this life, George opined, "*Es ist so die richtige Mischung aus Grandhotel und Zigeunerzelt.*" [This is just the right combination of grand hotel and gypsy tent.]

Despite the fact that four people occupied the not very large house, harmony reigned. Dr. Schlayer recalled a conversation on October 30, 1931, about how George, Frank, and she should answer one of Kempner's letters. George suggested, "*Aber wir wollen ausmachen, dass wir gegenseitig übereinander nichts Schlechtes, sondern immer nur Gutes berichten wollen—dann seien alle geschützt.*" [We want to agree that we will not say anything bad about one another but only report good things—then all are protected.]

In addition to the Molino in Locarno, during the summers of 1931 to 1933 George also spent time at the home of Gerda von Puttkamer in Wasserburg. On one of these visits, Puma made some remark to him in praise of Dr. Kempner, whereupon George exclaimed, "Why do you all find him so special?" She replied, "We don't *find* him special. He *is* special."

One day in 1933, while driving George in Berlin, Dr. Kempner told him that he had lost his job at the Charité. George was initially furious, but after considering for a few moments, he said, "That's good. Now you can drive me everywhere." This remark might suggest that George's attitude toward the gathering Nazi threat was flippant, but he took it very seriously. Some early proponents of the Nazi movement had interpreted George's writings as sympathetic expressions of their own philosophy: disdain for democracy, respect for discipline and self-discipline, the necessary emergence of an elite to lead society toward its fullest potential. Quotations from his works were offered as a rationale for National Socialism, tarnishing George's reputation at the hands of some historians after World War II. Furthermore, several of his younger followers, initially taken in by Nazi propaganda, confused it with George's vision of a German spiritual rebirth. As his friends knew from per-

---

* Once in Wasserburg, where George stayed a few weeks in the summers of 1931–32 and for a shorter time in 1933, Puma's son Alexander Schlayer, then four years old, asked for a cigarette. George declared, "*Kinder rauchen nicht. Frauen rauchen nicht. Ärzte rauchen nicht. Nur Männer rauchen.*" [Children don't smoke. Women don't smoke. Doctors don't smoke. Only men smoke.]

sonal experience, George himself was distressed and alarmed by what he saw coming. According to Alexander Stauffenberg, when he and George crossed Lake Constance from Germany into Switzerland, George exclaimed, "At last one can breathe freely again!" Some years after the war, Dr. Kempner described a conversation he had had with George regarding his apprehensions about the Nazis:

> The president of the German Reich, Hindenburg, was an entirely "good, honest soldier." In 1933, he was over 80 years old. Because of his exceptional contributions, the current government gave him a country estate, tax-free for him and his successors. The family was very pleased, and Hindenburg thanked his benefactors politely.
>
> In May 1933, another man [George]—a 65-year-old "author," according to his passport—was offered a large sum of money. He was to use it to support gifted young people who wanted to work for themselves rather than engage in a profession. The amount was very significant, to be spent anonymously, without any report or accounting. Someone suggested that non-Aryan friends, or those who had to do with "degenerate art" or the equivalent and had therefore lost their jobs, could continue to receive their former salaries from these funds.
>
> As [George] recounted the offer to a young physician [Kempner], he walked back and forth through two rooms. In the young physician's room stood a large, gray, lacquered wardrobe with a mirror; a gray, lacquered shelf; and a similarly lacquered bed, covered with a fine, shimmering green silk cover. The young physician sat on the edge of the bed and said, "Well, that's very nice. We'll be able to drink even better wine." The man who had reported all of this suddenly stood before him and raised his finger. "I want to tell you something: if one accepts even five pfennigs from these people, one is lost!" [Unpublished recollection dictated by Kempner]

It has been claimed, in support of George's supposed sympathy with the Nazis, that he attended a government-arranged celebration of his sixty-fifth birthday, but this is not true. That birthday was celebrated over a small dinner with Dr. Kempner and a few other friends at the Boetticherstrasse house, as previously described, with Christa von Roebel serving as the "maid."

In a letter dated June 7, 1932, Karl Wolfskehl wrote to tell George that, troubled by recent disturbing signs of political upheaval in Munich, he had left Germany for Basel. George replied on June 11: "The general confusion is indeed great, ... nonetheless, in what concerns you personally, you seem perhaps to see too darkly." As Wolfskehl later learned, George is supposed to have said to those with him, "What I see I cannot tell you in full. But you will all still experience it and pay for it. And much worse is yet to come." (*Seekamp et al 1972 p 382*)

When George was leaving Wasserburg in the fall of 1933, on his way to Locarno, Gerda von Puttkamer urged him to be sure to include Wasserburg in his plans for the following summer. George responded, "Dear child, by then I will see the radishes growing from below." He must have felt that his end was near, as indeed it was. He died in the Clinica Sant' Agnese, Locarno, on Monday, December 4, 1933, at 1:15 a.m. On the evening of his death, his body was taken to the chapel of the cemetery in Minusio.

The last gathering of a large number of George's friends and followers took place at his wake on December 5th and his funeral the following day. Originally the funeral service had been scheduled for the afternoon of the 6th, but when two representatives of the Nazi government made inquiries indicating that they planned to attend, the ceremony was shifted to the morning to avoid their presence. Until his burial, the roughly twenty-five people who had assembled took turns attending the coffin in pairs. The mourners included Clotilde Schlayer, who had been with George since September and remained to care for him until the end; Kempner, who had directed his medical treatment; Robert Boehringer* and his brother Erich; Victor Frank; Ernst Kantorowicz; Ernst Gundolf; the three Stauffenberg brothers; Ludwig Thormaehlen; Karl and Hanna Wolfskehl; Georg Peter and Edith Landmann; Josef Partsch; Michael Stettler; and Wilhelm Stein, among others.

After the burial, Ernst von Weizsäcker, a German foreign officer in Switzerland and one of the two intended Nazi party representatives, came to George's grave and left a wreath tied with a ribbon bearing the Nazi swastika. When Clotilde Schlayer discovered it, she rushed off and returned quickly with an armful of roses with which she completely covered the wreath. It did not disappear soon; indeed, it remained long enough for the ribbon to become frayed. Two young men appeared at the Molino and asked Frieda if she could mend it. Frieda resisted, protesting that she was too busy—and later asked Schlayer whether she had done the right thing. Schlayer assured her emphatically that she had.

As it happened, Weizsäcker was one of those later prosecuted at the Nuremberg Trials by Robert Kempner. He first denied any role in the Nazi

---

* Boehringer and Berthold Stauffenberg were Stefan George's co-heirs and literary executors. Frank was also named, but he died in battle in February 1943. After Stauffenberg's death in 1944, Boehringer became sole heir and executor. In the latter role he sometimes solicited Dr. Kempner's and Dr. Schlayer's advice on the publication and preservation of George's papers, and on proposed writings on George by others.

atrocities, claiming that the foreign office was not involved. When confronted with his signature on orders for massive deportations of Jews to concentration camps, he said, *"Ich bin erschüttert!"* [I am badly shaken.] His son Richard, who later became president of Germany, testified at the trial that Weizsäcker would return home from his office in the evenings deeply distressed, obviously aware that terrible things were happening but seemingly unable to extricate himself. He had stayed too long in his post, hoping at first that he might be able to ameliorate the evil he saw being done. Weizsäcker's relatively light sentence suggests that he was found to be more of a weak man than an evil one. Years later, his great-niece, Heilwig "Zuzu" Eulenberg, who had developed multiple sclerosis, was a patient of Dr. Kempner's in the rice diet program.

The combination of Hitler's assumption of power in February 1933 and George's death in December brought about a critically changed environment. George's followers, like millions of others, were all in some way victims of the Nazi regime, and they had, in addition, lost their pillar of resistance to it.

Adolf Hitler had made his position on Jews abundantly clear long before he became Chancellor of Germany in 1933. As early as 1919, when he underwent a program of political education for demobilized soldiers that emphasized German nationalism and anti-Semitism, he so impressed his superior officers with his zeal in these matters that they asked him to respond to a letter from Herr Adolf Gemlich inquiring about the "Jewish question." He wrote as follows:

> Antisemitism of the emotional sort finds its final expression in the form of pogroms. Rational antisemitism, on the other hand, must lead to a systematic legal opposition and elimination of those special privileges which the Jews hold, in contrast to the other aliens living among us.... Its final objective must unswervingly be the removal of the Jews altogether. (*www.holocaustdenialontrial.com/evidence/p1103*)

He reiterated these sentiments many times in the years following, notably with the publication of *Mein Kampf* in 1926 (even more so in the 1927 "second book" of *Mein Kampf*, which was not published until 1945). Germany must be cleansed of Jews, he said, because they were the root of Germany's misery following World War I: through their "international conspiracy" they dominated international finance and were responsible for the war, the decline of national values, the rise of Marxism, and the pernicious "mixing of the races." The language employed in *Mein Kampf* is that of raw hatred: the Jew is "a maggot in a rotting corpse," "the spider that slowly sucks the people's blood," "a pack of rats," "a harmful bacillus," "the vampire."

On January 30, 1933, after a chaotic year of power struggles with Hitler's political base, the Nationalist Socialist (Nazi) Party, Field Marshal Paul von Hindenburg, the incumbent president of the Weimar Republic, finally named Hitler Chancellor. Hitler wasted no time putting his intentions into effect. The burning of the Reichstag, the German Parliament, on February 27, 1933, was a galvanizing event. Even before the fire had been extinguished, Hermann Goering—later one of Hitler's chief ministers—was loudly blaming it on a young Dutch Communist, whom they had arrested on the spot. Nazi spies in Holland had found among a group of disaffected young men with anarchistic leanings a not very intelligent 24-year-old, Marinus van der Lubbe. They lured him to Berlin, furnished him with Communist papers, and planted him in the Reichstag. When the building burned, the police seized the "culprit," who was tried, convicted, and executed. The police chief who oversaw this arrest was Rudolf Diels, whose help Robert Kempner's wife later sought to achieve his release from the Gestapo. The only people who had access to the Reichstag were Goering and his henchmen, and it is now virtually certain that they set the fire themselves. The whole event was created as a pretext for suppressing the Communists in Germany.

Those in power well knew that in times of emergency, when people are most frightened, they become most willing to surrender their liberties in return for "security."

Thus, on the very day after the fire, Hitler persuaded Hindenburg to issue a decree suspending civil liberties. Two weeks later, he obtained special authority to deal with the crisis. By this authority he established, first, the dreaded People's Court, which tried cases of purported treason behind closed doors with no appeal, and then the Special Court, for political crimes or "inside attacks against the government." On March 23, under the Enabling Act, Hitler became dictator of Germany, immune to any legislative or constitutional constraints. And on Hindenburg's death, in August 1934, the presidency was abolished and Hitler assumed the title of Führer. (*www/fff.org/freedom/fd05403a.asp*) The Reichstag fire was a typical Nazi strategy. As Robert Kempner wrote: "Arson and misleading maneuvers have always been a major instrument of the Nazis ... Always arson, arson, arson." (*R Kempner Catalogue 1995 p 50*)

In his rise to power, the main thrust of Hitler's actions was, of course, against the Jews. In April 1933, Propaganda Minister Joseph Goebbels launched an attack on Jewish businesses, with widespread looting and vandalism as well as boycotts. April 7, 1933, saw the enactment of the Law for Restoration of Professional Civil Service, which excluded non-Aryans from civil service as well as from teaching positions; an additional law banned non-Aryans from practicing law. Two weeks later, Jewish doctors were banned from practicing medicine. Throughout the spring, organizations of students, professors, and librarians compiled extensive lists of "degenerate" books. On the evening of May 10, crowds of zealots, marching and singing by torchlight, surged into libraries and bookstores all over Germany to seize the offending books, which they threw onto huge bonfires in the streets. On that one night more than 20,000 books were burned on the Berlin Opernplatz alone. Many were by Jewish authors, of course—Max Brod, Albert Einstein, Franz Kafka, Sigmund Freud, Franz Werfel, among others. But a surprisingly large amount of the proscribed literature was by non-Jews (Thomas Mann—who had a Jewish wife—Erich Maria Remarque, Rainer Maria Rilke) and included many non-German authors. Jack London, Ernest Hemingway, Sinclair Lewis, and Helen Keller were among the Americans banned—Keller because of her physical disabilities, in accordance with the German eugenics program. More constraints, large and small, materialized: orthodox Jewish men were forced to shave their ear locks, and Jews, while still permitted to enter public libraries, were no longer permitted to sit there, nor on park benches. Then, in September 1933, German Jews were deprived of their citizenship altogether.

Thousands of disenfranchised Jewish scientists and academics, as well as anti-Nazi political figures, sought to flee the gathering danger. Fides's father, Alexander Ruestow, a political scientist and violent anti-Nazi, went as a voluntary exile to Istanbul in 1933. Karl Wolfskehl left Germany in 1933, spent about a year in Switzerland, then moved to Italy, which for a time seemed to be a safe haven. After Hitler's visit to Italy in the spring of 1938 indicated otherwise, Wolfskehl emigrated to New Zealand, where he remained until his death. Dr. Robert Kempner, after his release from arrest by the Gestapo in March 1935, also went to Italy, and in 1939 came to the United States. Barbara Zielke had left Germany for Istanbul in the mid-1930s as tutor to the Salz children. Both Ernst Kantorowicz (1895–1963), who was Arthur Salz's brother-in-law, and Ernst Morwitz (1887–1971), who had also lost his job, waited until 1938 to emigrate to the United States, and Ernst Gundolf left Germany for England only in 1939.

The difficulties encountered by people fleeing Germany were compounded by those of creating a new life. Finding homes and jobs abroad was not a simple matter. In the 1920s, the United States had enacted a series of restrictive immigration quotas allowing fewer than 26,000 Germans to enter the country in any year. The stock market crash of 1929 reinforced the nation's resistance to a surge of immigrants seeking work. To be accepted for entry into the US, refugees had to show proof of employment with a guaranteed income for at least one year. The urgent plight of German intellectuals prompted the formation, in 1933, of the Emergency Committee in Aid of Displaced Foreign Scholars. The New York-based organization functioned as a sort of broker, contacting US universities to solicit faculty appointments for endangered scientists and scholars, and providing a two-year subsidy of salaries with funds from the Rockefeller Institute. In all, some 6000 displaced scholars and professionals applied to the Emergency Committee. Of that number, 335 were placed in teaching or research positions in the US. (*NY Public Library, Division of Manuscripts and Archives*)

Walter Kempner's position at the Charité Hospital was terminated in April 1933, a casualty of the anti-Jewish laws. In defiance of the laws, Otto Warburg gave him a position a few weeks later in his Institute for Cellular Physiology. Warburg, who was partly Jewish, was left undisturbed by the Nazis because he had Hitler's direct protection. After removal of a polyp, which was benign, from his vocal cord, the Führer developed a morbid fear of cancer, and he considered Warburg his personal cancer expert. At the Institute Dr. Kempner studied enzymatic butyric acid fermentation, but this position was terminated in December 1933. Stefan George, whose medical care Dr. Kempner had been overseeing from Berlin, suffered a stroke on November 26. Immediately upon hearing the news Kempner left for Locarno to attend to him, without any warning to Dr. Warburg. Exasperated, Warburg told Kempner that his position at the Institute was terminated as of January 1. Lydia Kempner wrote to Warburg (December 28, 1933) urging him to reconsider and reinstate her son. George, she explained, was like a father to Walter; furthermore, in the prevailing political situation, losing this position would cut her son off from any possibility of doing scientific work or supporting himself. Warburg responded in a very angry letter (December 29, 1933) that Walter Kempner had twice left the Institute without saying a word to him, a breach of discipline he could not tolerate, as it demoralized the other staff.

> I had expected, when I gave your son a position after he had lost his job at the Charité, that, through his industry and interest in the work, he would earn the respect of his colleagues, who welcomed him very warmly. The opposite has occurred, and so it is impossible to retain him.

By this time Dr. Kempner had already begun looking for work outside Germany. When he mentioned the United States as a possibility, George expressed his opposition to Kempner's being so far away and wondered whether he might find a position somewhere on the continent or in England. Dr. Kempner and his mother both bent their efforts to find at least a temporary solution; like many others, they assumed the Hitler regime would be short-lived. That intelligent persons, strongly anti-Hitler, could still be very naïve about the political reality is reflected in Clotilde Schlayer's remark to Dr. Kempner in a letter of January 31, 1933, the day after Hitler became Chancellor: "*Ihm ist wohl gleich mit Hitler, mir auch*" (I reckon Hitler doesn't matter to you; to me neither). The fact that Morwitz, Kantorowicz, and Ernst Gundolf were all still in Germany in 1938 indicates that they too could not have fully realized the danger posed by Hitler, and probably had anticipated his early downfall.

In November 1933, Johns Hopkins University offered Dr. Kempner a position on the strength of a recommendation from Otto Warburg, but he declined, reluctant to put such a distance between himself and Stefan George and, evidently, still not realizing the extent of his danger. After George died on December 4, 1933, Dr. Kempner tried, for a short time, to open a private medical practice in Berlin, but it was increasingly clear that he would not be allowed to practice medicine. On January 18, 1934, Dr. Lydia Kempner wrote to Dr. Otto Warburg:

> I would be very grateful to you if you would inform me whether the position in Baltimore that you had offered to my son in November is still open and whether you would be kind enough to intercede for him in this matter. I enclose a curriculum vitae and a certificate of his medical training. Furthermore, I would be very grateful if you would have sent to me a certificate concerning his scientific capacities and his activity in the institute. With these I would still like to make an effort on his behalf in Switzerland with several clinics and biochemical institutes, though without much hope.
>
> Could you give me some advice where one might possibly apply for a position in England, and would you be so kind as to give my son a recommendation there to take along? I hope you will pardon my repeated requests in view of the difficulties of the present situation....

It is possible that Dr. Kempner's mother also contacted people at the Rockefeller Institute in New York, most likely its director emeritus, Simon Flexner, whom she had met while at the Women's Medical College of Pennsylvania. On behalf of both of her sons, Lydia Kempner also made inquiries in Geneva through the *Comité International pour le Placement des Intellectuels Réfugiés*. Inquiries in Edinburgh and London were fruitless. Her efforts eventually resulted in two tentative offers for Dr. Kempner, one from Turkey and one from Palestine, neither of which he accepted.

Then, on April 10, 1934, Dr. Kempner received a telegram from the Emergency Committee in New York: *Possible opportunity medical school Duke University North Carolina stop Research facilities stop Stipend two years stop Cable reply George Baehr 2 West 45 Street.* Dr. Kempner wired back: *Very interested please send particulars about character of position amount of stipend date of commencement many thanks Kempner.*

George Baehr, a clinical and research pathologist at Mt. Sinai Hospital in New York, was also a pioneer in public health and a member of the first Scientific Advisory Board of the National Institutes of Health. He was very probably acquainted with Lydia Rabinowitsch Kempner—certainly professionally, if not personally—through her work at the Medical College in Pennsylvania and subsequently in tuberculosis research, and may have been included in her letter campaign to relocate her son Walter.

On April 18, Kempner received a letter from Dr. Frederic Hanes (1883–1946), then chairman of Duke's Department of Medicine:

> Through Dr. George Baehr of New York I am informed that you would like to have a position in one of the American Universities. The Emergency Committee in New York has indicated that, should you come to Duke University in Durham, North Carolina, a salary of twenty-four hundred dollars per year will be given you for two years.
> … [I]t is my intention to be in Germany about the first of July and if you are interested in this position I could arrange to meet you somewhere in Germany so that we might talk the situation over thoroughly … It would probably be most convenient to see you in Berlin.

Having already scheduled a vacation trip to Europe with his wife, Hanes planned to take some time in Germany to contact several people recommended by the Emergency Committee for new faculty hires. He and Dr. Kempner made an appointment to meet in Berlin. On May 3, 1934, Dr. Kempner wrote to Bergmann at the Charité:

> My request to you would be whether you would speak with this Professor Hanes when he comes to Berlin, for you can obviously achieve more for me in a conversation of 20 minutes than I myself during his entire stay there. At the moment the offer seems to me rather mediocre; the position that Warburg wanted to get for me in November in Baltimore was much better, judging from externals, but perhaps something will also come of it here.

Gustav von Bergmann also supplied a letter of recommendation (November 20, 1933), as required by Duke:

> From November 1928 until April 1933, Dr. Walter Kempner was associated with the II Medical Clinic under my directorship. As assistant

of the clinic he had independent charge of large wards and worked con-
tinuously with the very extensive material of the medical outpatient clinic.

If, in this certificate, I do not speak of his outstanding qualities as
a research worker, of his scientific achievements and publications, of
his methodological training, it is only because this will be done by
others and because my own judgment in these matters is already apparent from the above. This is primarily an appreciation of Dr. Kempner as a clinician.

With his extraordinary gifts, he combines true warm-heartedness
and therewith the capacity of sympathy for patients, and the readi-
ness for sacrifice; thus he possesses those characteristics in the moral
sense as well, that qualify him particularly for the profession of physician and clinician. He has a lively interest in clinical problems and has
acquired great experience in both the scientific and practical aspects
of internal medicine. It is not often that theoretic and clinical gifts are
so united as in the case of Dr. Kempner. He was, moreover, not only
very popular with the patients but also with his colleagues and the
hospital personnel. Dr. Kempner has a great working capacity and is
intensely industrious. He is an excellent teacher with the ability to
present difficult problems with terseness and precision and may be
designated as an experienced, superbly trained clinician.

The letter of recommendation from Warburg himself has been lost. That
he took Dr. Kempner back onto the Institute staff despite the ban on Jews,
however, and that he arranged for him to be offered an appointment at Johns
Hopkins, speaks eloquently for the Nobel laureate's high opinion of his protégé.

Dr. Hanes had another highly recommended physician to interview on his
trip to Germany: Dr. Siegfried Josef Tannhauser was a professor of internal
medicine at the University of Freiburg, then in his fifties, with a distinguished
career and several important books to his credit. In their initial interview,
Tannhauser asked Hanes where Duke Hospital's patients came from. Hanes
replied that most were from North Carolina, some from South Carolina and
Virginia. Evidently Tannhauser found this unimpressive, and their discussion
of Tannhauser's possible relocation to Duke went no further. Tannhauser subsequently took a position at Harvard.*

---

* When Dr. Kempner—by then quite famous—was at Harvard in 1947 to give an invited lecture about the rice diet, Dr. Tannhauser, who had spurned Duke for its provincial
patient base, was in the audience. After the talk, he came up to congratulate Kempner, who
had heard about the Berlin interview. Dr. Kempner asked him, "Do you see many patients

The interview with the 31-year-old Walter Kempner was more successful. Dr. and Mrs. Hanes arrived at the Hotel Kaiserhof in Berlin around July 1. They declined Kempner's invitation to stay at his mother's house on the Potsdamerstrasse but did visit him there, as Mrs. Hanes wrote (July 6), "The memory of your kindness, the roses, Potsdam[erstrasse], coffee and raspberries in your home among the first editions and treasures of Greece will be with us always." The Haneses missed meeting Lydia Rabinowitsch during that visit, as she was ill and kept to her room. She later sent them a note apologizing for her absence, adding,

> You can easily imagine it would also have been of great importance to me to speak with you about the future of my son, Walter Kempner. I personally wish very much that my son should go to America, where I myself started my scientific career at a time when it was impossible for us women to obtain leading University positions in Germany. My teacher, Professor Koch, who was at first not very pleased at my leaving Germany, provided me at the time with such good recommendations to his pupils ... that it was not difficult for me to make my way there. But perhaps that was easier then than nowadays.
>
> The last time I was in your country was in 1927, when I had a very nice invitation from the American Association of Prevention of Tuberculosis to take part in their meetings and to give some lectures in different places. I should be very glad if my son should have the opportunity to continue his medical and scientific work there.

As Dr. Kempner showed the Haneses around the city, the two men talked at length. Dr. Kempner stated that he was interested in coming to Duke, but only on three conditions: he needed enough laboratory space, a laboratory assistant, and three consecutive months' vacation. In recounting the story of this meeting years later, Dr. Kempner remarked on his youthful naiveté in holding out for special conditions when the stakes were so high. The urgent matter at hand for him and many others was simply to get out of Hitler's Germany alive. On the vacation issue Hanes demurred, pointing out that Dr. Kempner would have a number of holiday leaves at Thanksgiving, Easter, etc. But Dr. Kempner explained that he would be unable to get to Europe and back in that amount of time. Conversation on that topic stalled. A day later, however, Hanes came

---

from North Carolina?" "No," replied Tannhauser. "Our patients come from Massachusetts and Connecticut. Why do you ask?" "Because," Dr. Kempner said with a smile, "I have so many patients from Boston and Massachusetts."

back triumphant. "You will have your three months vacation in a stretch! I just got a wire from the University." Thinking it over later, Dr. Kempner decided that Hanes had misled him: he had made that decision himself.

After the Berlin conversations, which evidently were satisfactory to both parties, the Haneses left to resume their travels, but the two men continued to discuss by mail the particulars of Dr. Kempner's relocation to Duke. On July 4, Dr. Hanes wrote the chair of Duke's biochemistry department, Dr. William Perlzweig, to assess his interest not only in working with Dr. Kempner but also providing him temporary housing upon arrival. Dr. Perlzweig responded,

> It so happened that just a few days ago Dr. Baehr wrote me and asked whether we were still interested in placing any of the men in our laboratories. I answered in the affirmative, indicating a list of men in which Kempner's name was first. I shall be delighted if you succeed in getting him to come to us, and I shall certainly extend to him all the facilities of my department.

Dr. Kempner wrote Hanes about available research equipment, particularly the Warburg apparatus, developed at the Kaiser Wilhelm Institute, for the study of cell metabolism under varying conditions:

> Two thermostats are the least one needs because with only one it is even impossible to make simultaneous observations of two different temperatures. Of course, many experiments of a certain kind can be done with *one* thermostat (Mozart is said to have played the violin better on one string than others on four), but it is naturally easier to work with a complete outfit if it is possible to obtain it. If not, I will manage as best I can with one.

Hanes forwarded his inquiries promptly to Duke and on August 12 wrote that he had

> just received a letter from Duke saying that there is one Warburg apparatus there already. So I think maybe it would be better not to buy until we see exactly what's there.

Dr. Kempner and Dr. Hanes continued these negotiations over several weeks. In spite of his favorable assessment of Dr. Hanes, Dr. Kempner was still ambivalent about the projected move to the United States; he wrote to Bergmann about his reservations concerning "America itself and the distance, not only in kilometers, from the things and people with which one really 'lives.'"

Finally Dr. Kempner decided in favor of Duke and, on July 17, accepted Hanes's offer. In the correspondence that followed came a letter from Hanes, still in Germany, which contained a puzzling sentence: "Now, if you wish to return fifteen hundred marks of the money I left with you in Berlin, you may send it to me in Freiburg in bills." Dr. Kempner was baffled; Hanes had left him no money. Dr. Kempner's friends suggested that he simply write or telephone Hanes and ask about it, but Kempner reminded them of the strict postal censorship and government wire-tapping. Finally, it seemed simplest just to comply with the request; on August 14, 1934, Dr. Kempner put the money in an envelope with a letter and mailed it to Hanes in southern Germany. On reflection, he conjectured that Hanes was helping him circumvent the restrictions on Germans taking money out of the country.

Dr. Kempner sailed to the United States from Bremen on Tuesday, October 9, 1934, and arrived in New York on October 15. In New York, he met with several members of the Rockefeller Institute and then continued south. He arrived in Durham on October 18 to take up his position as the first research faculty appointment in Duke University's Department of Medicine.

# A New Home

Upon arriving in Durham, Dr. Kempner reported immediately to Dr. Hanes's office at Duke. Hanes welcomed him to his new post and, after some conversation, opened his desk drawer and took out an envelope filled with bills, saying, "You might like this back now." It was the dollar equivalent of the fifteen hundred Reichmarks Kempner had mailed him from Berlin. "How did you get this here?" Dr. Kempner asked. "Ask my wife," Hanes smiled.

Having learned that German citizens were permitted to take no more than the equivalent of $10 out of the country, and aware also that communications were closely censored, Hanes and his wife had conceived the idea of mailing Kempner a request to send them money ostensibly their own. It was Mrs. Hanes's idea to tape the bills inside the tail light of their car, where they crossed the border undetected. The funds, changed into dollars, were enough for Kempner to buy a car. Kempner was not without his own subterfuges in getting money out of Germany. When he crossed the border, the ordinary-looking set of keys he carried in his pocket were cast from melted gold coins.

Dr. Perlzweig (1891–1949) and his wife, Olga Marx Perlzweig (1894–1988), welcomed Dr. Kempner into his temporary quarters in their house. It was located in the prosperous Hope Valley neighborhood, not far from the Duke campus, on a pleasant leafy street edging a golf course. Dr. Hanes had requested this accommodation for Kempner partly because of the two scientists' common areas of interest but also because Mrs. Perlzweig spoke fluent German, and Dr. Kempner's English did not yet come easily. The Perlzweigs were happy to comply. "My wife and I agreed readily that we shall be glad to take him into our home and attempt to make life pleasant for him," Dr. Perlzweig had written Hanes, but he cautioned that Dr. Kempner would need to arrange his own transportation—"a cheap car or a bicycle (not so good in bad weather)"—and the living arrangement, he wrote,

> will have to be tentative in the sense that it will depend upon our getting along and liking each other well enough. He should feel free to leave us if he finds living with us unsatisfactory; and we should be free to find him another place, if he constrains us too much. In other words, it would be dangerous for both him and us to make a permanent arrangement for two years before trying it out first. *In any event,*

*we shall be very glad to see him through the first few months here* [emphasis his], and after that I am sure we can settle things nicely.... Finally, our present economic status is such that we cannot permit ourselves the luxury of maintaining a guest for more than one or two weeks. He will have to pay his share of the living expenses, which will amount to about $45 per month. He will have a comfortable room and bath, two meals a day and such other comforts of our home as we have ourselves.

The placid southern tobacco town of Durham, then with a population of 35,000, was a dramatic change for Dr. Kempner. In Germany, before the Nazis, he had pursued his scientific and medical work with eminent European scientists in an atmosphere charged with the excitement of innovation; his circle of friends included some of Germany's leading literary and academic figures. From Durham, he wrote to his mother (November 2, 1934):

There's little to report from here; it is all like a hare-brained idea, neither good nor bad, actually not at all real—a story from the entertainment section of a provincial newspaper written by a not too gifted author, suitable for reading at a bus stop.... [In the clinic I see] many Negroes and serious illnesses; my laboratory [is] two empty rooms and a table. My activity: breakfast, usually alone, at 8:45; a fifteen-minute drive through fields and woods in my newly purchased green Ford to the hospital, to read English articles in a very well organized medical library surrounded by strange pictures of generals, horses, and exotic fowl. Afternoons, 3:00 to 5:30, instructing students in the outpatient clinic. At 6:00, family dinner; after dinner, coffee, and then I go to my room (which I like very much). I have a mail box with a key that is actually not a key but two numbers, turn right then left.

On November 29, he wrote her, "Mostly I am alone, which weighs on my English language conscience, because I actually speak rather poorly. I think people understand me merely out of politeness and not from the meaning of my words." Judith Perlzweig Binder, in an unpublished reminiscence of Dr. Kempner's coming to her family's house and his early struggles to master English, wrote:

[Dr. Kempner] arrived in Durham secure in the knowledge that he would be able to communicate with the natives. His English was terrible, the vocabulary sub-basic, the grammar poor, the meaning obscured by an extraordinarily heavy German accent. WK resolutely hacked out his sentences as if clearing a path through jungle undergrowth with a machete.

In the beginning it seemed hopeless: every written sentence was simply translated from the thoughts he had formulated in German in his head. German sentence structure, German word order, German tenses, German idioms, Germanic tone.

In composing the hundreds and hundreds of letters to his patients, WK was helped by friends who corrected his English, restructured the sentences and offered suggestions about how best to express his thoughts. These letters were written, corrected, rewritten, revised, rewritten, revised again almost *ad infinitum* until WK was satisfied (sometimes an hour after the native English speakers were satisfied). In the process WK hammered out his own English prose style, striking deep into the roots of the language, owing nothing to any teacher and nothing to the English literary tradition.

Under these circumstances, a stunning display of linguistic fireworks was the last thing one would predict but it happened. The most amazing was a spectacular triple pun, produced on the spur of the moment. A very special baked ham was brought to the table. When the recipe was explained to WK, how before the ham was put into the oven it was covered with slices of pineapple, glazed with brown sugar and studded with cloves like little spikes, he gave the ham a piercing look and suddenly roared "PORCUPINEAPPLE!!"

Even in his first months at Duke, aware that Duke's two-year commitment to him could end in 1936, Dr. Kempner had an eye out for other positions in the US. In November 1934, and again during the holiday recess from December 22 to January 2, he made two "business trips" to Baltimore, New York, and Washington to establish contacts with persons who might be able to offer him a job. At the Rockefeller Institute in New York, he also talked with several people about arranging an invitation to the US for his mother in connection with her tuberculosis research. Surprisingly, given the scope of his mother's work and reputation, and her own connections within the Institute, his efforts were unsuccessful.

By December, all the equipment for Dr. Kempner's laboratory had arrived and been set up in good order. On February 18, 1935, Olga Perlzweig wrote to Dr. Kempner's mother:

To continue my report of him, he is very busy and works tremendously hard. For weeks, we went to the florist to fetch him all manner of leaves [for his laboratory investigation of plant physiology], but now he is concentrating on pine needles, so that is very simple. One only has to go a few steps behind or beside the house to collect an abundance of such materials.

From Dr. Kempner to his mother, February 20, 1935:

Again nothing special to report. I was very industrious these past weeks, nearly all days and evenings, also Sundays, with my manometers and pine needles. I hope with permanent results. [Investigation of] tobacco mosaic [disease] eludes my industry, so I am having to study normal plant physiology on this occasion, and it seems very interesting and congenial.

On April 24, 1935, Kempner's life in America changed with the arrival of his friend Clotilde Schlayer. With considerable behind-the-scenes maneuvering, Dr. Kempner had managed to obtain permission for her to join him as a technical assistant in his lab. (It should be noted that this was not a salaried appointment; she had private funds, in the form of monthly payments from a Cuban businessman repaying her father for a favor some years before. The position at Duke simply provided her the qualification to enter the country.) Key to Dr. Kempner's success in securing her appointment was the fact that she had used the Warburg apparatus in Professor von Bergmann's clinic in Berlin and had mastered its highly specialized application. Bergmann's recommendation and, especially, her publication, in 1935, on her research with the apparatus (C Schlayer 1935) were sufficient to secure Dr. Schlayer's entry into the US.

Dr. Kempner wished to avoid the impression that Dr. Schlayer's employment was based on personal friendship rather than professional competence. Probably for that reason, Dr. Kempner disclosed to no one their prior personal acquaintance, and when she arrived in Durham, they greeted each other politely at the railway station as strangers.* Not until the early 1950s did I, and others among his close colleagues, learn that they were lifelong friends; in a shipment of Dr. Kempner's books and letters and other personal effects from Berlin, we discovered books in which he and Dr. Schlayer had inscribed dedications to each other, dating from their student days.

These belongings had been preserved for Dr. Kempner and finally sent to him by Emmy Allard (1881–1953), a teacher in the high school attended by Clotilde Schlayer and Nadja Kempner. Through Nadja, she became a friend

---

* I know this from two doctors who witnessed that meeting. Dr. Schlayer later described how difficult it was for the two friends to maintain a formal pose after such a long absence.

and admirer of the Kempner family. After the death of Nadja and her mother, Lydia Rabinowitsch Kempner, Dr. Allard visited and maintained the family grave site. After the war, the flower vendor from whom she had often bought flowers for the graves told Robert Kempner that she had reported Emmy Allard to the authorities for tending the graves of Jews. He was furious, and worried for her; however Dr. Allard apparently suffered no consequences. Her longest-lasting friendship in this group was with Dr. Schlayer, who visited her on her trips to Europe. She also developed friendships with Christa von Roebel and Ruth Peschel.

On her arrival in Durham, Clotilde Schlayer quickly settled into work with Dr. Kempner. On April 29, 1935, she wrote their friend Robert Boehringer in Switzerland,

> We are really undisturbed in the laboratory the whole day—except for the teaching hours—not very different from how it would be if we were active in Germany or elsewhere. We make our own tea (with your tea from Christmas) in the afternoon on the Bunsen burner.... Altogether, tea times and walks are an exception; otherwise we really work.

Only a couple of months after Dr. Schlayer's arrival, they traveled together to Europe to be with Dr. Kempner's mother, Lydia, who was ill and failing. On August 3, 1935, she died with her son at her side, and in October Dr. Kempner returned to Durham. This time, instead of returning to the Perlzweig house, he took a room in the Washington Duke Hotel, where he stayed until he bought a house in 1941. Dr. Schlayer remained in Germany until the end of December, assisting Robert Boehringer with the publication of the correspondence between Stefan George and Hugo von Hofmannsthal. (*R Boehringer 1938*) Until the outbreak of war in 1939, she and Dr. Kempner continued to travel in the summers to Europe; he usually returned to the United States before Dr. Schlayer, who stayed behind to see her family and deal with financial matters. As it turned out, the trip in 1935 was the last time either of them ever saw Germany,* though they continued to travel to other parts of Europe. Before and during the war, Germany was too dangerous for Dr. Kempner; for Dr. Schlayer, an Aryan, it was less threatening. Both, however, felt that "their" Germany was gone. More precisely, they concluded that it had never existed, for Hitler could

---

\* With one brief exception: In 1990, Dr. Schlayer crossed the Swiss-German border at Lorch-am-Rhein for the few hours needed to divest herself of her Berlin house at Boetticherstrasse 15c.

never have prevailed in the country they had believed Germany to be. When Kempner recognized the situation, he felt deeply betrayed and declared to Judith Perlzweig that he would never set foot in Germany again—unless someone very close to him were desperately ill and needed him. If he should return, he said, he feared he "might shake the hand of someone who had been a murderer." When the Peschels visited Germany some time after the war and looked up Dr. von Bergmann, they reported to Dr. Kempner that their old mentor had deteriorated sadly and seemed feeble and deeply depressed. I suspect that another reason Dr. Kempner avoided returning was his reluctance to encounter such devastation in people to whom he had been close.

Dr. Kempner's work on cellular physiology flourished between 1935 and 1939. His interest in hematological disturbances continued, but opportunities for investigating such cases came slowly, since, by the nature of the disturbances, only rare patients were found in whom the metabolism of immature abnormal cells could be accurately measured. If enough normal cells are present, their metabolism may be sufficient to obscure the disturbed metabolism in the abnormal cells. Among the first papers he published from Duke was one on erythroblastic anemia (*W Kempner 1936a*), in which he demonstrated that erythroblasts (young nucleated red blood cells), like leukemic cells, require oxygen to live and, in the presence of oxygen, do not metabolize sugar as readily as cancer cells or dying white blood cells normally do.

A memorable feature of this study was the baby alligators that were imported into the lab as the best available source of nucleated red blood cells. Dr. Schlayer often carried them around in the pockets of her lab coat, and when one of the creatures started to crawl out she would simply push it back down. One day she noticed a technician eyeing her with some trepidation.

"Marvin," she said, "Are you afraid of these alligators?"
"Yes, ma'am."
"But Marvin, they are much more afraid of you."
"That's it, ma'am," he replied. "And that's just why they'll bite me!"

Dr. Kempner and his associates published two more papers on the respiration of immature white cells. (*Kempner & Gaffron 1939; W Kempner 1939e*) In 1936, Dr. Kempner turned his attention to phaeohaemin, the enzyme involved in the oxygen metabolism of plants, which turned out to be identical to one of the two enzymes in animal metabolism. For this study, he examined parts of a variety of plants found in his new American environment, including plums, daffodils, oleander, and pine needles. Some of these—tobacco plants, Spanish moss—must have seemed quite exotic to him. He also continued his studies on the effects of inflammation. Prior to Dr. Kempner's early research on inflammation in Berlin, only grossly visible changes in inflammation (cell migration, redness, swelling, etc.) had been identified. His work elucidated the physiological changes of inflammatory response: decreases in oxygen, sugar and bicarbonate concentrations and increased lactic acid and acidification. Now Dr. Kempner was ready to investigate what these changes actually do to the cells—including malignant cells—of the organs where they occur.

Between 1935 and 1939 he and Dr. Schlayer (as well as Dr. Ruth Lohmann in Berlin) had conducted studies on the physiological effects of oxygen deprivation. In "Effect of low oxygen tension upon respiration and fermentation of isolated cells" he stated

> I have found a marked effect on respiration of variations of oxygen tension in micrococcus candicans, staphylococcus aureus, pseudomonas pyocyanea, Escherichia coli, monilia albicans, human erythroblasts and leucemic leucocytes, red blood cells of fowls and alligators, and young green plant cells (pine needles). The dependence of the respiration upon oxygen tension is greatest in the youngest cells and is influenced by physical and chemical changes in the cell medium such as pH, $CO_2$ concentration, and bicarbonate content. (*W Kempner 1936c, p 149*)

In a second paper, "Effect of oxygen tension on cellular metabolism," he said,

> The oxygen tension at the surface of the human or animal cell is determined by an equilibrium which results from the oxygen consumption of the respiring cell and from the oxygen supply to the tissue fluid surrounding the cell.... There are many diseases in which various kinds of injuries to various parts of the body cause disturbances of oxygen supply to the tissue fluid of one or many organs, e.g., mountain sickness, coronary occlusion, embolic and inflammatory processes, marked anemias, Raynaud's disease and so on. The primary phenomenon in these various diseases is always the same: lack of oxygen, and a subsequent fall in the oxygen tension at the surface of the cell. The clinical symptoms vary according to the function of the cells affected. (*W Kempner 1937, p 339*)

Kempner's observations on how oxygen deprivation affects cells underlay the basic concept leading to the rice diet. To put it in simple terms, the kidney requires oxygen for the metabolism of nutrients; if its oxygen supply is reduced by disease, a diet requiring less metabolism should ease the burden on the compromised kidney and compensate for its abnormal function. Several articles related to his idea were published under his guidance by his associates. (*Schlayer 1935, 1936, 1937; Lohmann 1931, 1934, 1938*)

The most important investigations for the development of the rice diet concerned the effects of hypoxemia on kidney cells. Until the 1920s, the kidneys' bodily function was thought to be limited to excretion. It was known that ammonia, a substance important in acid-base balance, was excreted by the kidney, but it was not demonstrated until 1921 (*Nash & Benedict 1921, 1922*) that the kidney actually produced ammonia, rather than simply removing it from the blood stream. In 1933, Krebs *(Krebs 1933)* established that the kidney produced ammonia by deaminating amino acids. Dr. Kempner found that ammonia production by the kidney was markedly inhibited by low oxygen tension. His experiments demonstrated

> that cessation of the chemical function of the kidney is not necessarily due to anatomical destruction but can be caused by a temporary change of the [oxygen] concentration in the cell environment. Lowered oxygen tension in the kidney reduces the aminoacid deamination with corresponding ammonia formation to a fraction of the normal rate…. Blood and tissue acids reaching the kidney as sodium salts, and normally converted there into ammonia salts, are now, due to the inhibited renal ammonia production, excreted into the urine as sodium salts; the blood bicarbonate drops, uremic acidosis ensues. But since the inhibition of deamination of aminoacids by lowered oxygen tension is a reversible reaction, the original rate of ammonia production is reëstablished with the rise of the oxygen tension to its physiological level. Transient uremic acidosis is thus explained as a result of the reversible inhibition of the deamination of aminoacids in states of renal anoxemia. (*W Kempner 1938b, p 118*)

Some years later, describing the effects of the rice diet on kidney disease, Dr. Kempner said of his early kidney studies,

> If in the course of a disease, renal tissue is destroyed and replaced by a scar, obviously the only metabolic reactions to be found will be those of scar tissue and no longer those of the kidney cells. (*W Kempner 1946, p 358*)

Disturbances in the cellular metabolism may take one of three forms, he reported: (1) normal, or undamaged, cells metabolize in an abnormal environment; (2) damaged cells metabolize in a normal environment; or (3) damaged cells metabolize in an abnormal, or damaged, environment.

Dr. Kempner's letters home to Germany, addressed to his mother but circulated, at his request, among his friends, reported on this work as well as on other aspects of his life in America. He expressed continued satisfaction with his surroundings, describing walks in the woods, occasional games of table tennis with his hosts—including their daughter Judith, who was then thirteen years old—and horseback riding a couple of times a month. In 1935 Dr. Kempner also initiated a literary venture with Olga Perlzweig to translate Stefan George's poetry into English. She demurred at first, saying that she would prefer to work on Rilke, but Dr. Kempner was, of course, persuasive, and she agreed to his proposal. As they embarked on the work her enthusiasm grew, and soon they were meeting almost daily, debating each word, each phrase. When Dr. Kempner moved out of the Perlzweig household after several months, he continued to return for lunch, primarily to continue his collaboration with Olga. Clotilde Schlayer became an active participant after her arrival in Durham, and, in the fall of 1938, a new collaborator, Dr. Ernst Morwitz, joined the project.

Ernst Morwitz (1887–1971), a prominent judge and a member of Stefan George's circle, was in imminent danger from the Nazis not only as a Jew but also for his political views. He even took the precaution of keeping cyanide on his person, in case of arrest by the Gestapo. On Morwitz's behalf, Dr. Kempner contacted Felix Frankfurter, Abraham Flexner, and Franz Boas, urging them to help. The records do not indicate what, if anything, they were able to do, but Dr. Kempner finally persuaded Mr. Charles W. Peppler in the Duke Divinity School to invite Morwitz to give a series of lectures. Morwitz came to the United States in October 1938, just before the *Kristallnacht*; his mother and sister, unable to escape, died in Germany. As a poet and translator himself, he became an important new member of the George translation project. When Dr. Kempner and Dr. Schlayer became increasingly busy in the laboratory and clinic, the burden of translation shifted to Dr. Morwitz and Mrs. Perlzweig. In 1943 an unfortunate incident soured Morwitz's relations with Kempner and Schlayer. Apparently disheartened by his financial dependence—housed with a friend of Dr. Kempner's, his lecture series for the Divinity School completed, his hopes for a teaching position unfulfilled—Morwitz, without consulting the others, sold the rights to a selection of George translations to a publisher for three hundred dollars. The published book (*Valhope & Morwitz 1943*) bore the names of Ernst Morwitz and Carol North Valhope as editors—the latter a *nom de plume* for Mrs. Perlzweig that Dr. Kempner had playfully invented based on the Durham neighborhood where she lived: Hope Valley, North Carolina. Dr. Kempner was distressed by Morwitz's betrayal, not least because the translations were incomplete, still rough, and an inadequate representation of George's poetry. After this unpleasantness, Morwitz left Durham and moved to Chapel Hill. There he secured a job teaching German at the University of North Carolina from 1943 until 1956. During the war, he compiled a German-English dictionary for the US War Department.

In better times, Morwitz relished telling stories of his courtroom days. A woman with five children, he said, came before him to sue for divorce, claiming that her marriage had never been good. When he pointed out that she and her husband nevertheless had had five children, she exclaimed, "All in fury, Your Honor. All in fury!" Once, after presiding over a hearing involving two sausage makers, Judge Morwitz asked them conversationally, "Which sausage is the best?" He said he would never forget their reply, as the two gentlemen exchanged a glance: "The best thing you can do, sir, is to eat ham!" Despite his humor, Dr. Morwitz was usually a rather silent and withdrawn man whose solitary figure glided around campus. The Duke students called him "The Phantom."

In 1946, again with Olga Marx Perlzweig, Morwitz published a translation of Gustav Schwab's book, "Gods and Heroes: Myths and Epics of Ancient Greece." (*Marx & Morwitz 1946*) In 1949, they produced a translation of George's complete poems, published by the University of North Carolina. (*Marx & Morwitz 1949*) In 1956, Morwitz left North Carolina for New York.

Dr. Kempner's relations with William Perlzweig were never as warm as with his wife and daughter. I think it likely that Dr. Perlzweig, who was a competent but not original scientist, was jealous of this brilliant, handsome, and self-confident young man. Not only had Dr. Kempner's early work already gained him a considerable reputation, but the translation project that he had introduced into the Perlzweig household was taking up a significant amount of Mrs. Perlzweig's time and interest

By the end of Dr. Kempner's two-year appointment to the Department of Medicine, there was no doubt of his extraordinary industry, his clinical and teaching skills, and the quality of his research. Dr. Hanes gladly extended his Duke appointment. Before the extension, however, and in anticipation of needing to find another job, Dr. Kempner had solicited recommendations in support of his search from Dr. Ludolf Krehl, with whom he had worked in Heidelberg, and from Dr. Martin Jacoby, an associate and friend of his mother, with whom Dr. Kempner had briefly worked. From Dr. Krehl, Bern, November 10, 1935:

> In 1927 Dr. Kempner was on the medical clinic in Heidelberg as assistant. He is an unusually sharp and intelligent person. I consider him particularly suited for solving scientific problems in the field of pathological physiology.

On October 26, 1935, Dr. Jacoby wrote:

Dr. Walter Kempner is known to me for years as an outstanding bacteriologist.... In Krehl's clinic in Heidelberg, in O. Warburg's institute for cellular physiology, and in V. Bergmann's clinic, he educated himself most thoroughly and excellently in the fundamental branches of the most modern biochemical methodology and biological procedures.

His judicious and lucid formulation of questions has led to fundamental results. We owe to him decisive advances in the area of the biochemistry of microorganisms and inflammation.

The gift[s] of research and teaching combine in him harmoniously. He is in a position to attract young colleagues and to develop them into researchers.

I am convinced that Walter Kempner will produce significant achievements in every position to which he is appointed.

Not surprisingly, his reappointment at Duke went through without a hitch, and these recommendations were not necessary. But then in 1937, the expiration date for his passport was approaching, and he applied to Germany for a new one. It was far from certain that a new passport would be issued to him, given his non-Aryan status. So, with the aid of Mrs. Perlzweig and with his characteristic head-on approach to problems, he devised an alternative document that he hoped would be acceptable in lieu of a passport, if necessary. First, he wrote out an affidavit of identity and nationality, which was notarized by Duke notary Judith Farrar, whose authority was certified by Mr. Crabtree, Clerk of the Superior Court in Durham County, who in turn was certified by the Secretary of State of North Carolina, who, finally, was certified by Cordell Hull, the Secretary of State of the United States. Mrs. Perlzweig then carried this document to Washington and collected visas from the consulates of Holland, Belgium, England, France,* Switzerland and Italy. Whether this unique and painstakingly assembled document would have served its purpose will never be known, because at the last moment an official passport arrived from Germany.

Until their voyage in 1939, Dr. Kempner and Dr. Schlayer traveled each summer to Europe, five trips in all, to reunite with friends. In Switzerland, they saw Robert Boehringer and Lydia Kerr, a friend through whom they received their mail while traveling. They met Emmy Allard, Ruth Lohmann, Christa von Roebel, Mercedes Gaffron, and Fides Ruestow at various times and in various places—mainly France and Italy. They also saw Bobby Lucy-

---

* The French Consul at first demurred, saying, "If this gentleman gets into trouble, who is going to pay for it?" After some talk, however, he approved the French visa.

Scott, who had given Kempner English lessons before he left Germany (and who probably knew the von Roebel family). They tried to persuade Ernst Gundolf and Ernst Morwitz to leave Germany, but neither did until circumstances forced them to in 1939 and 1938, respectively. In the fall of 1938, Fides Ruestow accompanied Dr. Kempner on his return to the United States. On Clotilde Schlayer's return passage a few weeks later, she sailed on the same ship as Ernst Morwitz, but he was withdrawn and depressed and they had little contact.

When Dr. Kempner visited Robert Boehringer in Geneva in 1938, Boehringer urged him to return to America immediately, as war seemed imminent. Dr. Kempner decided to trust his luck and did not cut his trip short; as it happened, Chamberlain's agreement with Hitler in Munich put off the war for about a year. The following summer, he and Dr. Schlayer took their customary vacation in Europe, traveling separately to visit friends. A sense of foreboding hung everywhere, and by late August both were persuaded of the urgent need to leave while it was still possible. There was an extraordinary coincidence: Dr. Schlayer in Switzerland and Dr. Kempner in England each decided to call the other at the same moment. Their calls, placed simultaneously, overrode the telephone linkup—they found each other already on the line before either phone had rung—and the call was never charged to either of them. Agreeing that immediate departure was essential, they gave up their reservations for a sailing on the Cunard Lines and hurried to book the earliest possible passage, which was on the Viking Lines' Kungsholm, leaving from Göteborg, Sweden, on September 1. They were first told that no space remained, then that there was only one berth available, which they declined. Finally, with much talk and a little cash, they obtained third-class tickets, each sharing a space with three or four other war refugees. On the day of sailing, while the two sat on a bench in the center of Göteborg waiting for the hour of embarkation, a plane flew low overhead and its payload of paper floated down into the air around them. The leaflets, printed in Danish, bore the stark headline, "*Krigen begyndt: Warszawa bombarderet*" ["War begins. Warsaw bombed."]. Kempner and Schlayer departed on the last scheduled passenger ship to leave Europe. They would not return to Europe until 1950. In March of that year Dr. Schlayer attended her parents' golden wedding anniversary in Spain. Dr. Kempner returned a few months later.

At Duke, Dr. Kempner continued his research on oxygen tension and its relation to cellular function. He also taught medical students in clinical rounds and classes. One day in 1939, running into Professor Perlzweig in a hallway, Dr. Kempner asked him, "What can you tell me about this Cold Spring Harbor Symposium?" Perlzweig replied with a sardonic smile, "Oh, that's a very prestigious meeting. Scientists like us would never be invited to it," whereupon Dr. Kempner pulled out the invitation he had just received to present his research there. The invitation was a mark of considerable prestige and proof of high professional regard for the quality of Kempner's work in cellular physiology, from his early research with Warburg and at the Charité Hospital to his later work at Duke. In some circles he was known as "Oxygen-Tension Kempner." His milestone presentation to the 1939 Cold Spring Harbor Symposium, entitled "The Role of Oxygen in Biological Oxidations," provoked a favorable and lively response. He began by disputing one of Warburg's ideas:

> All observers agree that there is no true connection between the real oxygen tension with which the cell is actually in equilibrium and the rate of respiration.... (*W Kempner 1939c, p 269*)

The main reason why Warburg missed the role of oxygen tension, Kempner explained, was that many of his experiments were conducted at zero degrees centigrade or under other unphysiological conditions. In briefly summarizing his own experimental results, Dr. Kempner stated:

> We have to substitute for Warburg's all-or-nothing theory of respiration the law of direct role of oxygen tension as a determining factor of the rate of respiration....
>
> Decrease of oxygen tension in animal tissues might explain the incidence of pathological conditions, [such] as that of reversible uremic acidosis, which one should attempt to counteract with high oxygen tension treatment. In contrast to this, diseases caused by bacteria whose main source of energy is respiration, should be treated by attempting to lower the oxygen tension in the affected organ. (*W Kempner 1939c, p 283*)

Expressed in less technical terms, organ function depends on oxygen supply. If the oxygen supply is lowered—by high altitude or injury, for example—the organ will not function normally. Lack of oxygen to the heart may cause pain, as in angina, or death of tissue, as in a heart attack. Warburg believed that cells respond simply to the presence or absence of oxygen, regardless of tension level, but Dr. Kempner had observed that the response was highly dependent on the degree of oxygen depletion. (I used to explain it to my patients like this: it doesn't make much difference whether you're run over by a 40-ton truck or a 35-ton truck; it may, however, make a great deal of difference if it's only a quarter-ton truck.)

Shortly after the 1939 Cold Spring Harbor conference, Dr. Kempner began treating kidney and hypertensive patients with his radical dietary regime and soon was achieving startling results. To continue patient treatment, he needed to obtain a North Carolina medical license. He had already made his initial move to apply for citizenship in 1938, his decision bolstered by growing awareness of atrocities in Germany, and he became a naturalized citizen on June 3,

1941. The State of North Carolina, however, had never issued a single license to a foreign-born physician and showed no signs of doing so, despite Dr. Hanes's petitions on his behalf. Having ascertained that several other states did grant licenses to foreign medical graduates and also had reciprocity with North Carolina, Dr. Kempner sent inquiries to Kansas, Vermont, New Hampshire, and Maryland. On May 6, 1942, he was interviewed in Concord, New Hampshire, but apparently some mandatory papers never came through and he did not get clearance to take the state board examinations. We have no documentation of his transactions with Kansas and Vermont. Maryland, however, accepted him as a candidate and scheduled his examinations for June 9–12, 1942, in Baltimore.

The examinations were a challenging proposition, requiring him to write on highly technical subjects in a "foreign" language. To prepare for all eight subjects in which he was to be examined, Dr. Kempner had a book compiled of questions from prior National Board examinations, along with the answers written out in English. He learned the answers by heart. Many evenings, several of us would meet at his house after dinner, taking turns to ask the questions and correct his answers. Dr. Schlayer demonstrated her fantastic mental powers, easily memorizing both the questions and answers faster than Dr. Kempner. One evening when Dr. Kempner did not know the answer to a question on breech delivery, someone said reproachfully, "Dr. Schlayer knows the answer." He replied furiously, "Dr. Schlayer's mind works differently!"

When the time came, he traveled to Baltimore for his board examinations with another Duke candidate, Dr. Hans Loewenbach, a refugee from Hitler, who had been relocated to Duke's Department of Psychiatry. In Baltimore, Loewenbach suddenly developed cold feet and said, "We could go back to Durham and come another time." Dr. Kempner replied, "I've paid thirty-five dollars for my train ticket, and I'm going to stay!" "Sometimes, Kempner," Loewenbach exclaimed, "you're really ridiculous!"

Dr. Kempner passed the examination, and on July 17, 1942, he received his Maryland medical license. When he asked the NC Board of Medical Examiners about licensing by reciprocity, however, he ran into an obstacle. Dr. W. D. James wrote him on September 14, 1942:

> I am returning your application … It is a strict ruling of the Board of Medical Examiners of North Carolina that each applicant for license must be a graduate of a Grade A medical school of the United States or Canada.

Hanes intervened on his behalf, and on December 4, 1942, Dr. James wrote to Hanes, "I will be very glad to present Dr. Kempner's application to the Board along with your letter of recommendation. I will do my best to inform the Board of Dr. Kempner's ability as you related it to me."

Hanes not only backed up Kempner's application to the Board, he accompanied him to Raleigh for his Board interview in the spring of 1943. Hanes used to tell a nice story about that meeting, at which Dr. Kempner became the first foreign medical graduate to receive a North Carolina medical license. The Board members were all practitioners from various small towns in North Carolina, with no connection to Duke, and they had little enthusiasm for foreigners. They did not discuss with Dr. Kempner any medical problems—Dr. Hanes having already filled them in on Kempner's outstanding background and qualifications—but rather wanted to find out about this 40-year-old stranger with the thick accent. At the end of several confusing questions, they asked him, "Where, in your opinion, is the best medicine practiced—in Germany or the United States?" Dr. Kempner's answer was, "I have always been accused of being arrogant and conceited, so I will tell you, since I am now here, the best medicine now practiced in the world is in North Carolina." The Board member who had asked the question, a genial, elderly doctor, slapped his knee and laughed, "You are all right! You are our man!"

Once licensed by North Carolina, Dr. Kempner became a member of the American Medical Association and was eligible for board certification in internal medicine, which he finally received in June 1946. Dr. Kempner's naturalization as a US citizen qualified him for service in the US Army, and in 1942 he decided to enlist. He was not accepted, however. His draft cards for May and November 1942 give his classification as 2A (occupational deferment). Dr. Hanes told him in no uncertain terms, "No matter what you do, I will keep you out of the military."

# Neu Dahlem

From the provisional security of his two-year appointment at Duke University, Walter Kempner began working energetically to secure safe passage from Germany to the US for his friends. Before the war and immediately after it ended, as he became increasingly well established, he used any available leverage to find or create the jobs that enabled refugees to enter the United States, as he had done for Clotilde Schlayer. He sought the help of influential people to provide affidavits and to intervene as needed on their behalf. He helped his brother Robert to come when his position in Italy was increasingly threatened; in return, Robert's political connections were of great help as Walter brought over his friends after the war. To those who hesitated in the face of the uncertainties of life in America, he said, "You are better off with two dollars in America than with your job, house, and savings in Germany."

In December 1934, as the Nazis were confiscating her family's publishing house, Edit Ullstein Glaser fled Berlin and visited Dr. Kempner for several weeks, to investigate the possibility of relocating to Durham. (After a brief marriage ended in divorce, she continued to use her married name.) While in Durham she made job inquiries on behalf of her friends Ruth Lohmann and Ernst Peschel, without results. Finding Durham a suitable place to settle, Glaser went briefly to England to see her brother and then emigrated in 1935 to Durham. She had earned a degree in social work in Berlin in 1928, and in America she resumed her studies, receiving her masters degree in psychology from the University of North Carolina in 1938. She applied for positions as a social worker at Duke and as a German teacher at Elon College (now Elon University), not far from Durham. Neither materialized, but she eventually became a research analyst for the state unemployment office in Raleigh, where she worked for more than twenty years.

Her father, Hermann Ullstein (1875–1945), remained in Germany until 1939, when he escaped to New York. There, the only work this accomplished and formerly powerful man could find was as a janitor. While carrying out his duties he managed to publish occasional essays on the political situation in Germany and a history of the family's publishing dynasty. (*Ullstein 1942*) Before leaving Germany, he had written a book on advertising, published in Switzerland probably because German firms would no longer handle books by Jews. (*Ullstein 1937*)

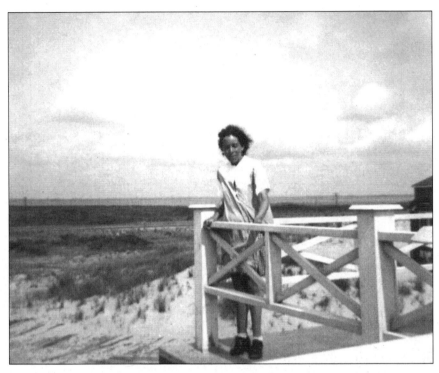

Figure 19. Edit Ullstein Glaser, probably in the late 1920s.

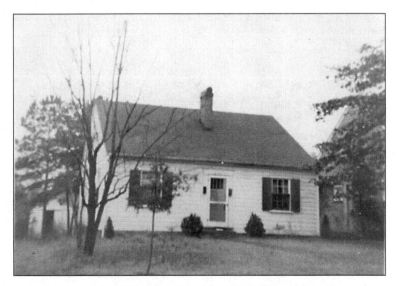

Figure 20. Edit Glaser's house at 2110 Wilson Street.

For a time after her arrival Mrs. Glaser stayed in the old Washington Duke Hotel, where Drs. Kempner and Schlayer both lived; in March 1938, she bought a modest house at 2110 Wilson Street, and she managed to have some of her furniture and part of her library shipped from Germany. Other household furnishings and possessions went to her brother and mother in England and, after her mother's death, more made their way to Durham. At her little house she served occasional teas and Sunday lunch to Dr. Kempner and his friends. To the children on Wilson Street, Mrs. Glaser was known as "the cookie lady," someone they could count on for a warm welcome and a cookie when they stopped by. In the early days she raised chickens in her back yard, and she kept Dr. Kempner well supplied with eggs—interesting, given his subsequent strong dietary principles. She must have had in mind his reminiscences about the early days in Heidelberg when money and food were scarce. On those occasions when he could obtain a few eggs, in his hunger he would sometimes break them against a wall and eat them on the spot, raw. One of Mrs. Glaser's favorite recollections was of the first time she entertained Walter Kempner for lunch at her house in Grunewald, a fashionable suburb of Berlin. Early in the meal, she was called away from the table to take a phone call. In her absence Gertrude, the housemaid, brought in the roast. The telephone conversation grew lengthy, and by the time she returned from her call Kempner had cleaned the platter and the housemaid had already taken it away. His hostess resumed her seat and asked Gertrude to please bring in the dinner. The poor maid didn't know what to say.

When Dr. Kempner returned from Europe in 1938, he was accompanied by Fides Ruestow. She entered the country with a visitor's visa and moved into the house at 2110 Wilson Street with Edit Glaser. Miss Ruestow enrolled as a student at Duke, with a concentration in humanities; she also took chemistry for her required science course. In 1940, as the situation grew ever grimmer in Europe, she was informed that her visa would no longer be renewed. She petitioned for a reversal of the decision and permission to stay in America, citing as her reasons that, first, her father was an exile from the Hitler regime, and, second, if she were to return to Germany her own anti-Nazi views would place her in danger. She further stated that when she came to America she had no intention of staying permanently, and that she still planned to return to Germany after Hitler's fall. Her petition, supported by an affidavit from Dr. Kempner along with letters from his patients, was successful, and by the time America declared war Fides Ruestow was employed by Duke in the Department of Physiology. In 1946 she transferred to Dr. Kempner's laboratory, where she worked until 1975 doing electrolyte determinations. Miss Ruestow lived at 2110 Wilson Street until 1948, when she bought a little house a few blocks away, on Stroller Avenue. This house was situated on a long, narrow piece of land which

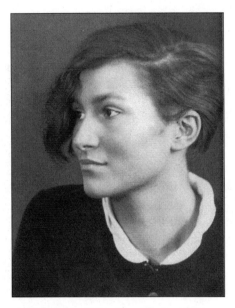

Figure 21. Fides Ruestow, ca. 1930.

she turned into an outstanding rose garden, bordered with magnolia trees. Dr. Kempner enjoyed visiting her on her porch overlooking the garden. She became a naturalized citizen in 1950, but remained nostalgic for the country of her birth.

Barbara Zielke Schultz, another pre-war arrival, came to the United States with Dr. Kempner's help in 1937, along with her husband, Hans Stefan Schultz (1905–1984). He was a relative of both the Henkell champagne family and Joachim von Ribbentrop (1893–1946), Foreign Minister of Germany from 1938 to 1945 and later convicted of war crimes in the Nuremberg trials and hanged. As a young man, Hans Stefan had worked his way to this country as a coal-stoker on a freighter and spent a year studying at Williams College. After his return to Germany, he obtained a PhD in classics from the University of Berlin in 1931 and, later, a degree in German literature. In 1937, he considered his chances of employment in the US better as a professor of German than as a classicist. His first position was teaching German literature at Skidmore College; later he taught at the University of Chicago, and published several articles on Stefan George and other German writers. While he was at Chicago, Barbara Schultz worked as a research assistant in the university's art department and in the catalogue division. In 1966, when her sister Christa became ill, Barbara Schultz moved to Durham to be with her. Her husband retired from Chicago and joined her the following year.

Another notable arrival in 1938 was Ernst Kantorowicz (1895–1963), an eminent historian at the University of Frankfurt who resigned that position in 1934 in order to avoid being forced out by the Nazi government. Although each was an admirer of the other's accomplishments, Dr. Kempner and Kantorowicz never knew each other well personally, and Dr. Kempner played no role in his immigration. He came to have particular respect for Kantorowicz, however, because of his courageous stand during the McCarthy era. As a member of the faculty at the University of California, Kantorowicz gained national attention for his refusal to sign the loyalty oath imposed on American academics. He wrote an impassioned manifesto on the matter, "The Fundamental Issue: Documents and Marginal Notes on the University of California Loyalty Oath," which was privately printed and circulated. His views on this crisis in American democracy coincided perfectly with those of Dr. Kempner, who urged all of his close associates to read the paper. Some excerpts follow:

> What the fundamental issue is has been obvious to me from the minute the controversy started. Perhaps I have been sensitive because both my professional experience as an historian and my personal experience in Nazi Germany have conditioned me to be alert when I hear again certain familiar tones sounded. Rather than renounce this experience, which is indeed synonymous with my "life," I shall place it, for what it is worth, at the disposal of my colleagues who are fighting the battle for the dignity of their profession and their university....
>
> From whatever angle one may look at the academic profession, it is always, in addition to passion and love, the conscience which makes the scholar a scholar. And it is through the fact that his whole being depends on his conscience that he manifests his connection with the legal profession, as well as with the clergy, from which, in the high middle ages, the academic profession descended and the scholar borrowed his gown. Unlike the employee, the professor dedicates, in the way of research, even most of his private life to the body corporate of the university of which he is the integral part. His impetus is his conscience. Therefore, if you demoralize that scholarly conscience, that love and passion for research and for teaching, and replace all that in a business fashion by strictly defined working hours, prescribed by the "employer," you have ruined, together with the academic profession, also the university! Only the culpably naïve ignorance on the part of the malevolent regents, not knowing what a scholar's life and being is, could venture to break the back bone of the academic pro-

fession—that is, its conscience—in order to "save the university," nay, to dismiss a scholar for that very conscience which makes him a scholar.

Folly, like the spirit, bloweth where it listeth. All that stupid destruction of genuine values and valuable human beings is carried on for the sake of a historical demand the utter folly of which has been attested to nationwide; it has been attested to also by the professors' new company, the gambling-house nude, who takes her loyalty oath deposed in a champagne glass for the customers. Folly knows no limit. We can only pray with Erasmus: *Sancte Socrates, ora pro nobis!*

Kantorowicz left Berkeley as a result of this controversy and spent the rest of his academic career at the Institute for Advanced Study in Princeton, where he wrote his powerful and influential treatise on medieval legal and political history, *The King's Two Bodies*. (*Kantorowicz 1957*) The book's subject is the conflict between the office and the individual: the king, as king, can do no wrong and cannot die, but as a person he is of course both fallible and mortal. Shakespeare touches on the dilemma in *Richard II*.

Kantorowicz was a renowned gourmet as well as historian, and the story was told that once, en route from his house in Princeton to catch a train, he suddenly asked the friend driving him to stop the car, turn around, and drive him back to his house. He had forgotten something. Asked what, he said, "My truffles." He added, "Do you ever travel without your truffles?"

Hitler's invasion of Poland and the outbreak of war in Europe put a stop to emigration from Germany. After the war, however, the flood of refugees from Germany resumed. The battered country, divided into occupied zones, suffered from the devastating aftermath of war. People had lost their friends, their families, their homes; there was not enough food or fuel, nor was there a foreseeable opportunity to resume their vocations. Dr. Kempner resumed his efforts to bring friends and colleagues to America.

Ruth Lohmann had visited Durham briefly in 1935, seeing patients with Dr. Kempner and meeting Dr. Hanes. She had returned to Germany and been trapped there by the war. In 1946, her first opportunity to leave the country again, she and Ernst Peschel, whom she had by then married, came to Duke with the help of Dr. Kempner and his brother Robert. They both went to work for Dr. Kempner. Initially they moved in with Dr. Schlayer, who had left the Washington Duke Hotel in 1940, rented for a year at 909 Knox Street,* and then in 1941 bought a house near Mrs. Glaser's, at 1503 Virginia Avenue. Dr. Kempner at the same time had

---

* Dr Schlayer took great pleasure in saying the address: "Nein, oh Nein!"—in plain English, "No, oh no!"

bought the house next door to her, number 1505. (These two houses were said to be the last two built in Durham before the United States entered the war and building materials became unavailable.) I believe that Dr. Kempner stayed in the hotel as long as he did because he could not let go of his conviction that the situation in Germany would be short-lived and afterwards he could return home. He simply refused to believe that the Germany of his youth would tolerate the Nazi regime. But after the *Kristallnacht*, in November 1938, and Hitler's annexation of Czechoslovakia gave his hope the final blow, he began to look on America as his permanent home and gradually arranged his life accordingly.

Dr. Ernst Peschel worked in and directed Dr. Kempner's laboratory until the early 1960s. Starting in 1958, he saw private patients at Duke, especially those suffering from kidney disease. He was instrumental in establishing the dialysis unit there in 1957, the year he and Dr. Kempner were visited by Dr. Willem Kolff (1911–2009). Kolff, a Dutch physician, developed the dialysis machine during World War II in his efforts to treat soldiers suffering kidney failure. He first published a report on this work in 1944, and in 1947 he visited major medical centers in the United States to promote his new machine. At that time Dr. Kempner had tried in vain to persuade Duke to invite Kolff to lecture. When he finally arrived ten years later, I feel sure that their discussion focused on dialysis. In the late 1960s or early 1970s, Dr. Peschel left Dr. Kempner's staff to devote himself to practicing medicine, first at Duke, where in 1970 he became Professor of Medicine, and then, upon his retirement in August 1971, in private practice in Durham. He retired completely in the mid-eighties.

Dr. Peschel was an exceptionally fine musician; in fact, he had once considered making music his profession. When he chose medicine instead, he supported himself through medical school by playing cello. He owned and played a rare Grofiller cello, made in Venice around 1710. He must have purchased it after arriving in the United States, as it would surely have been difficult for him even to possess such an instrument in Germany, let alone get it out of the country. I remember that, after a performance at Duke, the Budapest String Quartet came to the Peschels' house and joined him in playing chamber music. For many years, he played privately with members of the North Carolina Quartet (affiliated with the University of North Carolina in Chapel Hill), and he occasionally participated in their public performances.

Ruth Lohmann Peschel worked initially with her husband on statistical analyses of patient data for Dr. Kempner's scientific publications; she later served as a patient counselor and, after taking qualifying examinations for a North Carolina license, as a physician. In 1949–50, the Peschels acquired a small prefabricated house on a lot purchased by Dr. Kempner at 2306 Pershing Street, just around the corner from Dr. Schlayer's and Dr. Kempner's houses on Virginia Avenue.

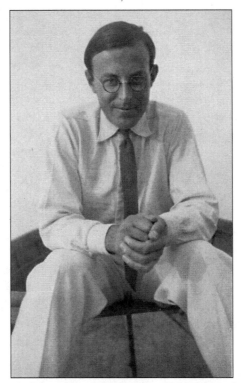

Figure 22. Ernst Peschel, probably taken shortly after his arrival in the US in 1947.

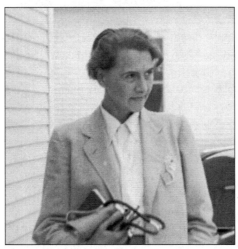

Figure 23. Ruth Lohmann Peschel, probably ca. 1950s.

Mercedes Gaffron and Christa von Roebel, both of whom had visited Dr. Kempner in Durham and had arranged to emigrate to America in the fall of 1939, were, like Ruth Lohmann, trapped in Germany by the war. After the war, however, with the help of the Kempner brothers, they made their way separately to the US. Thanks to her Peruvian passport, which allowed her to enter via Belgium and Peru, Mercedes Gaffron arrived in 1947. She, too, moved into 2110 Wilson Street and stayed there until 1961, when she bought a house close by, at 1612 Maryland Avenue. She lived there until, in 1989, she moved to the house previously occupied by the Schultzes, at 1500 Alabama Avenue. In 1948 she joined the psychology department at Duke, where Dr. Kempner—by that time running one of the most prosperous clinical practices in the country—set up a fellowship for her which financed her work from 1953 to 1969. In a letter to Dr. Kempner (July 4,1963), the department chairman, Dr. Karl Zener, wrote:

> Your continued and increased support of the work of Dr. Gaffron in our department has enabled her in the last few years to bring closer to a level of concreteness and comprehensiveness suitable for fuller public communication her highly original contribution to the psychology of visual art. The increasing recognition of her work among psychologists is a matter of real gratification to myself, my colleagues, and the university.

In her research on visual perception, Gaffron determined that the eye takes in images in a rising curve from lower left to upper right. (*Gaffron 1950a*) Deeply interested in art, she had published a book on Rembrandt's etchings (*Gaffron 1950b*) demonstrating that when Rembrandt created the printing plates for his etchings he had organized his pictures spatially on the plates themselves, not allowing for the fact that the image would be reversed in the printing process. Dürer, by contrast, had taken the reversal into account. In 1962 she received a grant from the Ford Foundation to observe and photograph Egyptian architecture and reliefs. She spent seven weeks in Egypt, accompanied by Karl Zener (1903–1964) and Friedrich Krauss (1900–1977). Krauss was an architect with whom she and Dr. Hanna Ruestow shared a house in Munich for many years; Zener was her collaborator, along with Donald Adams (1902–1971), on much of her research in perception. These two colleagues became good friends as well. In 1969, by which time Dr. Adams had retired and Dr. Zener had died, Mercedes Gaffron reduced her active involvement in the psychology department and joined Dr. Kempner's staff as a patient counselor, taking over work which Dr. von Roebel had been doing until illness forced her retirement. Dr. Gaffron continued with Dr. Kempner until the late 1980s.

Christa von Roebel, who did not arrive until 1949, acquired another little prefabricated house just across the street from the Peschels, at 2303 Pershing.

She obtained work at Duke in bacteriology and gynecology, her salary funded from 1949 to 1965 by a fellowship set up for her by Dr. Kempner. Dr. Bayard Carter, then head of the Department of Gynecology at Duke, had seen her operate on a visit to Leipzig and was very glad to have her in his department; he called her "a most skillful surgeon." Later she joined Kempner's staff as a patient counselor.

Thus, between Kempner's arrival in 1934 and 1950, a considerable number of German émigrés, drawn to Durham by their connection to Walter Kempner, established their own little community in a single Durham neighborhood. They were highly educated people who shared not only language and nationality but their love of European culture. They had shared as well, of course, the horrific situation in Germany and the loss and endangerment of their own family members and friends. To an extent, they must have felt isolated in a provincial Southern town with its mixed feelings about foreigners, Jews, and especially—during those years, certainly—Germans. It cannot have been easy for the post-war arrivals. They had been through the war, they had been in the occupation. The Peschels had been interned in a displaced persons camp. Dr. von Roebel made a harrowing escape through the salt mines near Leipzig from the Russian Zone into the American Zone, whence she was able to emigrate to America. Their English was not good; the food was strange, the housing was unfamiliar. They found American-style built-in closets, for example, a mysterious and poor substitute for European wardrobes. North Carolina's summer humidity and heat were intolerable. These realities only served to draw them closer together.

There was a significant difference between the circle of friends in pre-Hitler Germany and the group as it coalesced in Durham. In Europe, the young people had been well connected, well educated, and, for the most part, wealthy; they had taken for granted their freedom and mobility, pursuing their own broad interests in different, if overlapping, circles, and they had not been particularly clannish. Uprooted in America, by contrast, they became a real community, into which I and several other American-born friends and colleagues were welcomed.

Among themselves, the émigrés referred to their little neighborhood as "Neu Dahlem," after the Berlin suburb of Dahlem around which their lives in Germany had centered. Walter Kempner's house at Potsdamerstrasse 58a, Lichterfelde, where his mother continued to live, was only about a fifteen minute walk from the Dahlem house at Boetticherstrasse 15c, where he later lived with Clotilde Schlayer and where Stefan George made his Berlin headquarters in 1928–1933. The Warburg Institute was in Dahlem, and Ruth Lohmann, Edit Glaser and Mercedes Gaffron also lived near Dahlem in the neighboring suburbs of Grunewald and Zehlendorf. During the post-war partition of Ger-

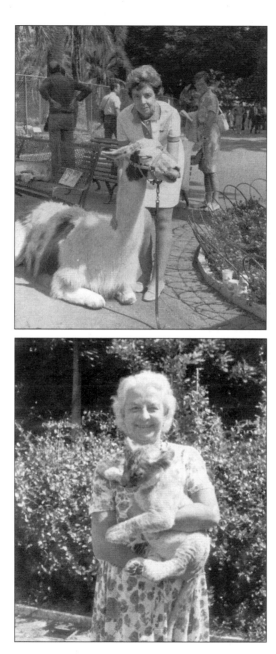

Figures 24 & 25. Charlotte Tilley poses with a llama, and Christa von Roebel with a lion cub, at the Rome Zoo, on one of the summer vacation trips in the early 1960s.

many, these areas were part of West Berlin. (In 2005 I visited both Boettich-erstrasse 15c and Potsdamerstrasse 58a; from the outside the houses and their neighborhoods seemed basically unchanged from former times, with very lit-tle evidence of wartime disruption.)

While some of the émigrés, like the Ruestows and to some extent Mercedes Gaffron, persisted in their hope of returning to Germany and never truly ac-cepted America as their home, Dr. Kempner and Dr. Schlayer felt themselves truly transplanted and embraced their new life. Dr. Schlayer loved American magazines; she even wrote letters to columnists. I remember one in particu-lar. A woman had complained to Ann Landers that her husband messed up her beautifully tidy, sparkling house, strewing his possessions everywhere, not keeping to any mealtime schedule, and so forth; she asked if she could justi-fiably confine him to a couple of rooms. Dr. Schlayer fired off a response: "The woman should be confined to one room! After all, it is his house. He paid for it, and he should throw *her* out if she doesn't like his ways." The idea that some-one must be tidy enraged her. She read a great deal of American poetry, good, bad, and indifferent. She sang American songs and, in the last years, she sang American, English and Scottish songs more often than the German ones. She loved clothes and always dressed up for holidays: red, white, and blue on the Fourth of July; green for St. Patrick's Day. She once bragged that, through cre-ative use of accessories, she had not worn the same outfit twice in a year.

When I first visited Durham in late March 1939, Dr. Kempner and Dr. Schlayer were still living in the Washington Duke Hotel, and Mrs. Glaser and Fides Ruestow were living in the small house at 2110 Wilson Street. Ernst Mor-witz must also have been at 2110 Wilson. From my first meeting with them, I became a frequent visitor in Durham, coming on college vacations or during the summer as often as I could. Until I graduated from Swarthmore in 1941, I stayed in Hope Valley with my friend Judith Perlzweig, who like me was fas-cinated by Dr. Kempner and his circle. We took meals with them occasionally at 2110 Wilson Street, which at that time served as their informal gathering center. We happily volunteered to help with chores and clean-up, and some-times, much less enthusiastically, helped catch Mrs. Glaser's chickens and clip their wings to prevent their flying the coop.

Christmas of 1941, which I spent in Durham, was a muted holiday; the radio played constantly with news of the war in Europe. But the circle of friends maintained a festive air, exchanging gifts and food and admiring each other's decorations. At least one Christmas tree was filled with lighted candles. Mrs. Glaser served her *bunter Teller*, a platter filled with a variety of cookies and candies. Ju-dith and I gave Dr. Schlayer a record player, her first since arriving in the US, and a recording of the Beethoven Violin Concerto. It was a great success.

Following my graduation in 1941, I spent a year taking courses at New York University—primarily, under Dr. Kempner's influence, pre-med courses in anticipation of medical school. I was also swayed by Dr. Kempner to include courses in Greek and geology. During that year, I managed a few visits to Durham. As Judith was by then in graduate school at Johns Hopkins, I stayed instead with Dr. Schlayer in her house. Fuel was being rationed, and I remember one visit when the house was so cold that standing water froze. Dr. Kempner, always the most stoic among us, told me that, in order to conserve heating oil, he directed the heat from a lamp onto his thermostat to "fool the house into thinking it was warmer."

In 1942, I finally moved to Durham, where I first lived in a boarding house not far from Drs. Kempner and Schlayer, who by then were established on Virginia Avenue. I took a job as a statistician at North Carolina State University in Raleigh. The job served its purpose of paying the rent, but I learned a good deal more than I wanted to know about the factors determining optimum egg production in hens. While there I also enrolled in a course in cellular anatomy. I took many meals with Dr. Schlayer, who was a fine and versatile cook, and helped her with household chores. Some time during 1943, I finished at NC State and began full-time employment in Dr. Kempner's laboratory on the fourth floor of Duke Hospital. My primary job there was to take blood samples from patients and to analyze them for sodium, chloride, and potassium content; I also made some determinations on urine samples. In mid-1944, I moved into Dr. Schlayer's Virginia Avenue house, where I remained until transferring to Chapel Hill to begin medical school in 1945. From there I commuted to Durham—a twenty-minute drive—on weekends and occasionally during the week, to continue working in Dr. Kempner's laboratory. On the weekends I stayed with Dr. Schlayer. In those days, the medical school at Chapel Hill was only a two-year program, so in 1947 I transferred to Johns Hopkins medical school to complete my studies. In 1949, after receiving my MD degree, I came to Duke for a year's internship and two years as assistant resident in the Department of Medicine. In 1952 I joined Dr. Kempner's staff full-time as a physician.

For many years Dr. Schlayer fixed weekday lunches for Dr. Kempner, his secretary Charlotte Tilley, me, and sometimes other members of the staff. She wasn't always happy with the conversation at her table, however, which she felt was excessively concerned with patients and clinical matters. In the mid-1950s, Dr. von Roebel or Dr. Gaffron took over the cooking duties once or twice a week. Mrs. Glaser, whose job in Raleigh prevented her from joining the group on weekdays, gave Sunday lunches to which the Peschels and others came. In the 1970s the Schultzes took over these Sunday lunches. As pre-

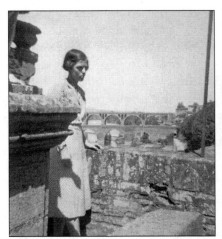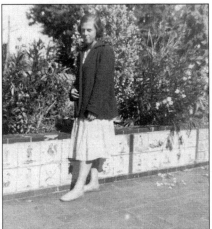

Figures 26 & 27. The author on a summer trip, ca. 1950. L: Southern France.
R: At Clotilde Schlayer's childhood home in Torrelodones, Spain.

pared by all these volunteer chefs, the communal meals were wonderful occasions; the culinary standard was high and European, the conversation equally
so—lively discussions about current events, literature and culture. The group
habitually celebrated birthdays, Christmas, and other major holidays together.
There was a basic incompatibility, of course, between our indulgence at the
table and the developing goal that brought us all together: working with Dr. Kempner to achieve good health through a strict diet. Over time, as this incompatibility grew harder to ignore, except for special occasions the group modified
its diet to conform more closely to healthy nutritional guidelines, if not the
strict rice diet—much to the initial consternation and disapproval of the chefs.
However, with great ingenuity, they found ways to create healthier variations
of the menu without seriously compromising its appeal.

The members of this group were able to leave behind their lives of considerable privilege and luxury and to embrace in Durham new lives of modesty and
simplicity, doing their own gardening and housework while continuing to pur-
sue the pleasures of the intellect. We never tired of hearing Dr. Kempner's stories from school and university days, and he in turn was a tireless storyteller. His
tales were studded with his early experiences of theater and opera and with
lengthy recitations from literature. As a student in school he had studied both
Greek and Latin for a number of years and had regularly attended theater, where
he became familiar with the classic German repertoire. One day, he told us, a teacher
had told the class in response to some disruptive behavior, "You will stay after
school." Walter Kempner, in his role as class leader, said, "We can't stay today. We

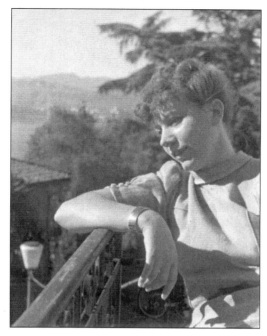

Figure 28. Mercedes Gaffron in Switzerland, 1941.

have the theater!" The teacher exclaimed, "*Schweinehunde brauchen nicht ins Theater!*" [Swine-dogs have no need of theater!] Theater and opera were important to him from childhood; as described earlier, he achieved an early triumph as producer, director and star of a school production of *Antigone*, in Greek.

Sometime in the 1950s or 1960s, Dr. Kempner received the gift of a phonograph, on which he played his favorite operas for us. Among them, I remember Mozart's *Don Giovanni* and *Marriage of Figaro* and Offenbach's *Orpheus in the Underworld*. Several chaises longues resided permanently at the corner of Virginia Avenue and Pershing Street, available for a little sun-bathing just before lunch. There, on Saturday afternoons, Dr. Kempner and others would lie in the sunshine listening to the Texaco Metropolitan Opera broadcasts. It was clear to us that he knew the music of many operas very well. In later years, there was less music and more reading. He enjoyed having one of us read aloud to him while he rested. We read the works of Homer or Pindar in German translation, Shakespeare in English, and the German poets.

Clotilde Schlayer's twin brother, Karl (1900–1987), a physicist, remained in Germany at the war's outbreak; he had found a job in telecommunications, which allowed him to avoid political involvement. But when he and his second wife, Nora, were able to leave Germany in 1946 to attend a conference in

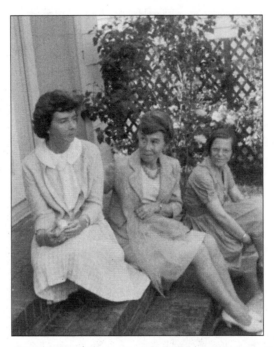

Figure 29. Charlotte Tilley, Clotilde Schlayer, and the author at
Dr. Gaffron's house at 1612 Maryland Avenue, Durham, 1962.

Switzerland, they took that opportunity to make their absence permanent and, following the conference, went to Madrid, near his parents' home in Torrelodones. He was not able to get a job there until 1950, when he found a position in the State Institute of Electronics.

Mercedes Gaffron's brother Hans (1902–1979), who, like Walter Kempner, had worked in Otto Warburg's institute in Berlin, was a biochemist with a particular interest in photosynthesis. In 1930–31, he had spent a year as visiting professor at the California Institute of Technology in Pasadena. In 1934, back in Berlin, he was arrested by the Gestapo but apparently was quickly released. In 1937 he came to the United States, with some financial aid from the Rockefeller Foundation, although his name is not included on the Emergency Committee's list of rescued scholars. In 1938 he took a research position at the University of California. He came occasionally to Durham to visit his sister Mercedes, and he and Dr. Kempner would have lively scientific discussions. Their father, Dr. Eduard Gaffron, was an ophthalmologist who gained renown in Peru as one of the few ophthalmologists then performing successful cataract operations in that country. Many of his grateful patients made gifts to him of pre-Columbian pottery and textiles, and he accumulated an important collection. On his death, part of the collection passed on to his children, who donated it to the Art Institute of Chicago and to the Duke University Museum of Art.

Fides Ruestow's sister Hanna spent 1938–39 in England as a pediatric nurse. In 1939, she returned to Germany to attend her grandmother's birthday celebration and thus fortuitously escaped being interned in England. She remained in Germany throughout the war, and from 1941 to 1948 was first in medical school and then in postgraduate training in Munich as a pediatrician. In October 1945, she received, in a letter posted through Geneva, the first postwar word from her father in Istanbul, where he had fled in 1933. She answered him with a lengthy account of how she and others had survived the war years; it is worth quoting extensively:

Dear Father,

Two weeks ago I received via Geneva the first news from you, and very soon thereafter a letter from Gertrude [her sister] from Hamburg, in which she writes that she too had heard from you. As you can imagine, we are very glad to know that all is well with you there, only we are very unhappy that we cannot yet give you any news. For you are much more uncertain about us than the other way around. I still do not know for certain whether and how this letter will reach you, but perhaps a possibility will present itself next week. In any event I want to have this ready.

First of all, at Felderfing and Königinstrasse we have all survived the war, and relatively well.... Impossible to go into every detail. Too much has happened since we were last able to write each other. But I will send you something of an account, and here for starters is a picture of the situation. For the past two months, the three of us are again, as before, living together in the little apartment in the Königinstrasse, Mercedes, Dr. Krauss, and I. Dr. Krauss appeared at the door one day at the end of August, dirty and tired. He had fought his way through from Kiel, having been discharged from the Navy, to which he had been drafted unnecessarily as a sailor (!!) half a year before the end of the war, through intrigues at the Hochschule. Since his arrival, we do practically nothing but provide for the necessities of the coming winter, about which we are very, very fearful, mainly because of Mercedes. So we comb the ruins to gather firewood, and Krauss saws, hacks, and hammers uninterruptedly. We installed stoves ourselves that we dug out of the debris of some friends' previous apartment. We repair doors, glaze defective windows with Rollglas, an emergency solution for which we are nevertheless very grateful, and construct the most extraordinary things to seal the windows.

We have now succeeded in furnishing one of our two large, light, and delightfully lovely rooms as a general winter living room—also still Mercedes' and my bedroom. It has turned out so well that all our visitors are enthusiastic and now leave even more reluctantly than before. To this I must add that, basically, we are once again living in the withdrawn fashion that we were once used to. This had changed utterly in the last months. In the horrible confusion of the bombings, our apartment, being in the cellar, had become something of an asylum for terribly many people who, when we were not actually sitting in the cellar, came in and out as if they considered it perfectly normal. Immediately after the end of the war we put a firm end to this, and now everything is more peaceful. I remind myself constantly how unimaginably fortunate we have been—I, personally, and all of us— in the small apartment in the Koeniginstrasse. During these past six years, we really lived together and were never alone. It was always peaceful, even when the bombings and everything connected with them were exhausting and turbulent. We helped each other as much as possible, and most of all we concerned ourselves as far as possible with sensible things, and so emerged from this war not too much dumber or worse. This we owe above all to Mercedes, who never allowed herself to be defeated and kept us all above water. But to imagine all of this, or even to articulate it so that it becomes imaginable, is hardly possible. Even though all sorts of unpleasant things will appear in this letter, I must also tell of those, because I am constantly aware how fortunate I was. I was able to study—even not knowing what the future would bring, especially with regard to money. But I hoped that I would be able to get somewhere, if already only through your position. We'll see.

But to return. Last April, the house in the Koeniginstrasse burned down to the second floor. The remainder could be saved, and our little garden—which was no more than a pile of burning rafters—came to life again through loving effort, and even now, almost in November, a sea of roses. Mercedes lies down a lot since last year, partly because of her knee, partly because of the constantly deteriorating stomach and intestinal situation, and general weakness. She works a lot, however, and during the past year has worked and written about things that, as soon as they are published, will certainly arouse attention [she published her Rembrandt book in 1950].

From 1 November on—since my studies have not yet been reinstated—I shall work for the military government to earn money, since,
like all non-Nazis, we all have nothing left. And Dr. Krauss's professorship for the history of architecture at the Technical College, which
was until recently not possible for political reasons, will be reinstated,
but will still take a while, like all such appointments. In the meantime, we have sold Mercedes' little car, at least to get through the winter, and can unfortunately not yet provide appropriately for the family
in Felderfing [Hanna Ruestow's mother and maternal aunt], who are
at the moment entirely without resources. Aunt Riele, however, gives
English lessons and is otherwise also very enterprising.

We moved out there at the end of the war, which was very good
because, from May on, Felderfing, a village of 1500 inhabitants, was
saddled with 3,000 former concentration camp internees, occupying
American forces, and, in addition, French troops who were billeted in
our house for three weeks on the march back to France. Three of them
lived with us, but five of them had to be cooked for all day. They
brought their own provisions, but the work was just as great, and
often it was not possible to cook the unusually good meals without
being challenged. This period was pretty terrible, and with all the
work would have been impossible had I, and partly also Mercedes,
not worked through from morning till evening.

As close as we were to Munich, we were unable to get news of how
things were during and after the surrender. There was a quarantine
for weeks in Felderfing because of typhus and typhoid, so it was late
May before we came back into the city—an adventure, because we
had no idea whether American Negroes or someone else was quar-
tered in our apartment. (We found it free and enchanting as always,
and were happier than ever.) That is to say, you would perhaps not
find it enchanting at all, for all the walls have cracks, some of the
doors are just nailed together, and suchlike. But with [*missing text*]
that is simply difficult. As for conditions in German cities, in this case
chiefly Munich and the impact there—that is entirely out of the question. I can only say that, as far as we can see today, Munich, despite
everything, is still Munich. At least, its character has not entirely been
lost, which is already a lot.

And yes, Felderfing: The two out there have been very affected by
developments: the continual work, which is always much too much for
them, and not least by their nutrition. In the shortest time, they have
become unimaginably thin, and also old. Aunt Riele was recently op-

erated on for a cataract, which did not go well. Fortunately, she will regain sight completely in the operated eye, but only after months. The other eye is so far half blind. Mother is recovering only with difficulty from a seven-week bout with intestinal flu, which has affected her terribly. In the summer, an acquaintance was there to help, like an angel from heaven, but needs to return now, of all times, to Austria, which is a big blow for them.

If only we had heat, but the only fuel is what we can forage for ourselves. Enough said. If you should find an opportunity to send something, do perhaps see if you could get some fat to the two in Felderfing. They can fend for themselves even less easily than we. We are hoping especially at the moment that the house in Felderfing will not be confiscated, which is not at all certain. That would mean that they would have to leave, perhaps within a few hours, abandoning the furniture and without any real place to go. In Felderfing, many Polish Jews are to be settled—and have to some degree been already. But right now we are thinking no more than 24 hours ahead, and try not to be too anxious about everything.

From time to time, in circuitous ways, mail from variously occupied areas makes it through, and so we have had news that Gertrude is doing relatively well. And, as absurd as it sounds, she will try to come on vacation. Aunt Hedi, who again tells us about all the rest of the family, says everyone has come back again from the front, and, although they had to endure a lot, all are glad and grateful. Unfortunately, there was terribly sad news, which they got only much later, that Aunt Else was struck by shrapnel from a grenade during the battle over Berlin. She died soon after, but without pain, thank God, and in the hospital. Dear Aunt Else—she never could have been taken out of Berlin, nor did she want to be, not even during the worst bombings. We are all terribly sad about it, and how dreadful it must be for you. The lady who helped us so nicely in Felderfing during the summer was a friend of Aunt Else's from last year and talked much and charmingly about her.

The news from here must seem to you to come from another world, and that is how it is. Nevertheless, we are thinking already and always of seeing each other again. We wonder what your intentions are, whether you are thinking in any way of coming back, if there were a professorship for you or other possibilities. I do not suppose that your plans or the situation here, however, make it likely that you would like to return. You certainly have people in Germany who would make inquiries for you, though I do not know what your relation to them is. Dr. Bauer wrote Mother that he had been imprisoned for months, but now he is doing well and wants to try to continue helping Mother. She is very happy about this, since she has been without money since March.

One sometimes paints silly fancies for oneself. Mercedes and I thought how well it would work out, when everyone returns, if you would take most of the Felderfing furniture and [Mother and Aunt Riele] would finally "retire" to appropriately smaller—and, for them, very much more comfortable—conditions. This is something that we have wished for ardently for the longest time, even though the two have become somewhat immobile and would have trouble initially getting used to the idea. This is still only an idea, but for you it is perhaps really important to be able to count on it, which you can under all circumstances.

It seems to me that I may not write much longer, otherwise no one will read this letter. If it works out as I hope, an American professor, who has been placed in Frankfurt but will be here from time to time, can take it. You may be able to reply to his address in Germany; it might also be possible to send something to, or through, him. He has already offered most kindly to help us with mail to and from America, but would that also work for Turkey, or via Switzerland? We shall see. The professor brought news of Mercedes' brother in Chicago, though we do not yet know anything directly from Fides, but we have written her. And that is the most important, for the moment. Whether the Gaffrons' house in Schlachtensee has, in the meantime, been more completely destroyed and whether the maid still lives remains unclear. It was already in such a state that one could not count on it any more, except as a burden. In addition, the most valuable part of the [Peruvian?] collection is certainly with the Russians and so in reality nothing is left. For [Mercedes?] in her state, this is particularly terrible; nevertheless, she is not too discouraged, because everything is uncertain and unclear.

Please do try as soon as possible to give me precise news and let me know your plans. One would like so much to learn more, and above all to make contact again. Maybe I shall find a way. I shall do everything. (The Red Cross at the present time doesn't work at all.)

Take good care of yourself and let us hear from you soon. Mother is trying also from her side to write you. Forgive me if this letter is somewhat confused. This is partly due to the circumstances, partly that I am under the influence of many pills, which alone make it possible to keep going. Within two weeks I have two totally infected teeth, of which one is already out. The other absolutely should be preserved, although it causes aggressive and continual pain. Recently, one's last powers of resistance seem to be losing out. One is completely without resistance to infections, and we hear the same thing everywhere. But let this be the last complaint. As I glance over this letter I note that there is no mention that, indeed, on an hourly basis, one is indescribably happy, first that these terrible years are over—and the attacks—for which one still often thanks Fate. But so it is. It is often more difficult to write about the most important things; nonetheless, these things exactly are clear to all and always in one's mind. You especially. For now, the very very best to you all, and of us more precise news soon.

Most warmly, your Hanna

In October 1951, Hanna came to Durham to visit her sister Fides and her friend Mercedes; the latter had emigrated in 1947. At this time she first met Dr. Kempner. From then on, while continuing to practice as a pediatrician in Munich until 1989, she returned at least once a year to Durham, where she worked with Dr. Kempner and his patients. In addition, she met Dr. Kempner and his friends in Europe. She introduced his nutritional principles to Munich, where she successfully treated several nephrotic children with the rice diet. Although Germany was still suffering economically from its defeat, it is worth noting that she was able to keep these nephrotic children on hospital wards for six months at government expense, which would not have been possible in this country. After retiring from her medical practice in 1989, she spent most of her time in Durham, staying with Dr. Gaffron in the Schultzes' former house on Alabama Avenue.

Elizabeth Gilmore Holt (1905–1987) was another person drawn into this circle and until her death was a good friend of both Dr. Kempner and Dr. Schlayer. A noted art historian, Dr. Holt taught at several American academic institutions, including Smith College and Duke, where she and Dr. Kempner were introduced, in 1935 or 1936, by Professor William Stern and his wife, Clara, German refugees relocated to Duke by the Emergency Committee. Once, when giving a lecture at Duke on the artist Käthe Kollwitz, Elizabeth Holt was astonished when a member of the audience presented her with a letter from Kollwitz. It was Fides Ruestow, who in 1926 had lived for a year with the Kollwitz family while studying photography in Berlin. After the lecture, the two dined together with Drs. Kempner, Schlayer and Morwitz.

Another member of the circle was Rosabel Coutts Eadie (1894–1981), wife of George Eadie, head of Duke's Department of Physiology. As early as 1936, Dr. Kempner and Dr. Schlayer visited the Eadies, who were neighbors of the

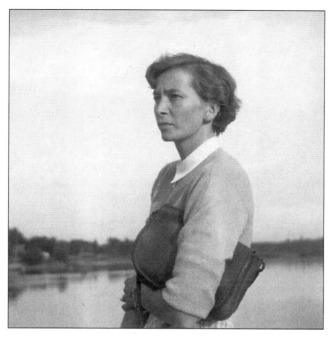

Figure 30. Hanna Ruestow, ca. 1960.

Perlzweigs. Mrs. Eadie had worked in Toronto with Frederick Bunting and Charles Best. Their Nobel-winning research introduced insulin to the treatment of diabetes. She had, in fact, witnessed the first insulin-induced hypoglycemic reaction: When she observed a patient, an elderly clergyman, trying to balance his socks across his toes, she reported his odd behavior, whereupon his blood sugar was tested and found to be too low. Mrs. Eadie began working with Dr. Kempner as a volunteer in 1942–43, taking blood pressures, talking with patients and relaying their questions and complaints to Dr. Kempner, encouraging their efforts to stick to the diet. Before going up on the wards she would often remark, "Now, I will go and build morale!"* With Dr. Kempner, she worked out going-home diets and instructed the patients on how to fol-

---

* As Judith Binder later recollected, in a letter to me, "Rosabel's great contribution was impressing upon the patients the necessity of following the diet exactly. In slow, measured, resonant tones, with an indescribable authoritative—not authoritarian—seriousness, entirely different from the bright, brisk, routine efficiency of the hospital personnel, and with her noble appearance, as of a sovereign disguised in a white laboratory coat, Rosabel, with her somewhat distant air, got through to the patients in a way that all the chummy 'moral support' practiced by others could never achieve."

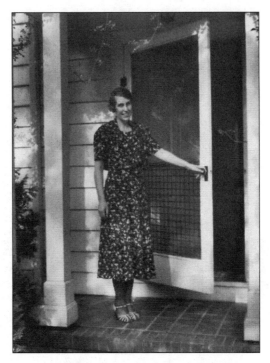

Figure 31. Rosabel Eadie, ca. 1950.

low the diet after leaving Durham, scheduled their return check-ups, and so forth. Her usefulness to Dr. Kempner's program greatly impressed Dr. Eugene Stead, chair of the Department of Medicine at Duke and founder of the Physician Assistant program; in fact, she might well be considered the prototype for the physician assistant's role. She was frequently among those invited to Dr. Schlayer's lunch table. In 1963, having reached the mandatory retirement age of 69, she retired from Duke.

Dr. Helen Starke (1918–1995) came to Duke as a medical student in 1938 and had courses with Dr. Kempner during all four years of her medical schooling. After receiving her degree in 1942, she joined the Duke house staff in internal medicine for a year, after which she became part of the house staff at the University of Rochester, New York. When Dr. Kempner presented his research on the rice diet to the annual meeting of the American Medical Association in Chicago in 1944—the historic talk which brought national attention to the rice diet—he invited Dr. Starke to assist with his poster presentation. While they were there, he persuaded her to return to Duke to join his staff as medical assistant, a position she held until 1953.

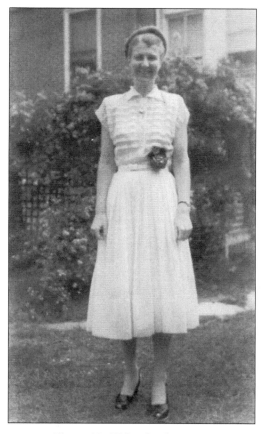

Figure 32. Helen Starke, 1953.

The two were good colleagues and friends, and their respect was mutual. However, although Dr. Starke received her most significant training from Dr. Kempner, she had also become well grounded in conventional medical practice both at Duke and at Rochester, which made her hesitate over some of Dr. Kempner's unusual medical procedures. For example, it was common practice at the time to search for a surgically treatable cause of hypertension by using special kidney tests that included taking x-rays after injection of dye into the arm. This procedure was safe, but was sometimes followed by another diagnostic test, a so-called retrograde pyelogram, that required injecting dye via the urethra and bladder, and this sometimes led to a kidney infection. Dr. Starke ordered the latter procedure on a patient, and Dr. Kempner, who felt the risk outweighed the benefits, countermanded the order. Dr. Starke protested, "But without it you can't make a diagnosis." Dr. Kempner replied, "Then I

shall treat the patient without a diagnosis." More than once, in patients unable to get sufficient nourishment by mouth, Dr. Kempner ordered intravenous
injection of a highly concentrated sugar solution, a procedure proscribed in
many hospitals because of potential damage to the vein. Dr. Starke (and later
I) gave these solutions reluctantly, but we learned from Dr. Kempner how to
administer the solution very slowly and avoid any injury to the vein. Dr. Kempner was also somewhat unconventional in his response to students presenting
a patient. They ordinarily started with the chief complaint, proceeded to the
family history and thence to the past history. Dr. Kempner, impatient at this
stilted method, at times would interrupt with a question. One student, irritated
at being thrown off his stride, said, "Should I give you the history, then, or do
you want it piecemeal?" Dr. Kempner said, "In this case, I would like it piecemeal."

In 1952, through the influence of a monsignor who was a rice patient, Dr.
Starke converted to Catholicism, took religious vows, and entered the Maryknoll order. In time, she resumed the practice of medicine as a nun. She and
Dr. Kempner maintained their friendship through correspondence for the rest
of her life. In fact, she returned twice to Duke to cover for Dr. Peschel and me
when we were on vacation.

In 1947, when Dr. Eugene Stead came to Duke to chair the Department of
Medicine, he queried his senior faculty closely to clarify the function and assess
the effectiveness of their staff. Most of the faculty were rather lukewarm in their
assessments. But when Dr. Kempner was asked about Dr. Starke, he said, "She's
completely different from me. When she has six patients to see, she spends an hour
or an hour and a quarter with the first one, and the same with the next one. She
is not the least bit hurried. Now I, I see the first one for a quarter of an hour,
and so on, and for the last one I take all my time." Stead asked, "Isn't Dr. Starke's
method better?" Dr. Kempner replied, "Of course it is. But who has such nerves?"

Dr. Kempner's long-time secretary, Charlotte Tilley (1929–1988) was an
important member of his circle. A native of Durham, she began to work with
him in 1946 when she was less than a year out of high school. She proved to
be indefatigable, with a keen instinct for organizational management and a
fantastic memory. We all relied on the skillful way she ran the office; Dr. Kempner prized her highly for her administrative skills and, over time, as a friend.
He gave her much credit for the success of the rice diet program's administration. I remember my first encounter with Miss Tilley. She was sitting across from
Dr. Kempner at his desk watching as he folded a letter to put it into an envelope. Without a word, she reached over and took the letter from his hands and
folded it herself, much more quickly and neatly than he. I was much impressed
by her calm confidence in her own skills, as was Dr. Kempner. In a letter of 1967

requesting her promotion, Kempner wrote, "She has the rare distinction that in all these years I have not heard a single complaint about her from any one of the literally thousands of people she had to deal with," and praised her "patience, modesty, unselfishness, and kindness." Miss Tilley was another participant in the daily luncheons. She and I became very close friends, spending a good deal of our leisure and vacation time together.

Katherine Ormston (1908–1995) first entered the picture as a patient in February 1948. She was referred to Dr. Kempner by Dr. Irving Wright, a well-known New York cardiologist, after every attempt to treat her extreme hypertension—including sympathectomy—had proved ineffective. She was an unusual patient for two reasons: first, for over six months on a strict rice diet her disease scarcely improved, the longest anyone had been on the diet without marked response. Second, and fortunately for her, she was an unusually motivated and enlightened patient; she had seen in her own family the tragic results of hypertensive vascular disease, and through her work with the Lasker Foundation in New York was knowledgeable about cardiovascular research. So, when Dr. Kempner told her that he thought she should persist with the rice diet for a very long time, but that she would need constant observation, she simply moved permanently to Durham, where she obtained a job at Duke. Not until almost four years after she began the rice diet did she make substantial improvement.* In the meantime, she held, for a time, the position of executive secretary of the North Carolina Heart Association.

She also joined Dr. Kempner's staff and made herself valuable in several ways. She instructed patients on the regime to be followed in Durham and, when it came time for them to return home, counseled them on maintaining their motivation and self-discipline. She was a good psychologist. I remember her conversation with one young man with hypertension, who protested that the restrictions of the rice diet would be very inconvenient in his social life, his bridge club meetings, etc. "Let me tell you, then, how things will be," she replied. "At a future meeting of your bridge group, someone will say, 'Two clubs,' the next will say 'Two hearts,' the next will say, 'Did you hear poor Maury had died? Three spades.'" The patient commenced the diet and followed it for over forty years.

Katherine Ormston wrote for and edited the bulletin of the Walter Kempner Foundation, established in 1949. Of her own illness and recovery she wrote:

> Most important to me personally, is the fact that since September 1, 1948, I have been steadily engaged in earning my own living, with only the usual vacations and holidays.... This work has required steadily

---

* Her interesting case is described in greater detail on page 160.

increasing activity and responsibility, long hours of work and considerable travel.... Looking back, it seems to me that my blood pressure decreased as my work and responsibility increased....

Best of all, to me, has been the consistent feeling of well-being. I
have, throughout the past five years, slept well each night (with no
medication whatever) and wakened with sufficient energy to carry me
through a busy day without difficulty. I am, in fact, living a normal,
busy, happy life; I just can't eat everything I'd like to have. Perhaps in
the future even that will be remedied. (*WKF Bulletin 1953 p 16*)

Bernice Krasne (1912–1989) first came to Dr. Kempner in 1947. At age 35,
her blood pressure, even under sedation, was 222/130, and she had a strong
family history of vascular disease. Under Dr. Kempner's treatment, she showed
an excellent response, and on returning to New York became an enthusiastic
ambassador for the rice diet treatment. Mrs. Krasne was well connected in
New York society, and she amused and entertained Dr. Kempner with her stories of a world with which he was little acquainted—and from which he drew
a number of very prominent patients. After her recovery, she worked as a volunteer for the United Nations, receiving and entertaining its high-ranking visitors, while adhering to her modified rice diet.

Over the years she made frequent follow-up visits to Durham, often for two
to three weeks, and the force of her ebullient personality leavened the atmosphere in the rice houses. She provided warm encouragement, giving the other
patients hope for their own recoveries, and she herself provided an excellent
example of a full and enjoyable life while following the rice diet. Her own case,
in fact, showed that, over time, one could gradually resume a minimally restricted
diet, as long as fat and salt were carefully controlled. She was able to maintain
her health on a diet of vegetables and cereals, to which, without detriment,
she gradually added small amounts of seafood, chicken, eggs, butter, and
cream. In 1955 she became a member of the board of the Kempner Foundation. In 1972, as vice president of the Foundation, she wrote in the Bulletin,

I myself, who was critically ill 25 years ago from extremely high blood
pressure with severe eyeground involvement and having a dire family
history of cardiovascular disease, made a complete recovery and have
enjoyed 24 and a half years of perfect health. I would not be alive
today if it were not for Dr. Kempner's research and its practical results. (*WKF Bulletin 1972 p 8*)

When the Germans invaded Belgium on May 10, 1940, Helen Mertens
(1910–1997) and her husband, Otto Rosenthal Mertens, were able to escape

to America, but their flight through France, Spain, and Portugal seriously compromised Otto Mertens's health. After a variety of operations and treatments in New York, he was told that the physician of last resort for him was Dr. Kempner, in Durham, from whom he first sought treatment in 1952. After this first visit, Mertens suffered a series of strokes, so he returned to Durham and lived in the Rice House on Mangum Street until his death in 1970. Helen Mertens maintained residence in New York to keep the family's chemical business going, but she visited her husband regularly, and felt particularly indebted to the kindness of Drs. Ernst and Ruth Peschel. In 1964, she bought a house at 1410 Alabama Avenue—next door, successively, to Hans Stefan and Barbara Schultz, Mercedes Gaffron, and Hanna Ruestow. With her considerable business skills and proficiency in German and French, she was of great help to Dr. Kempner and became a good friend and member of our community. (It was she who, on hearing Dr. Kempner's tale about the chocolate June bug, arranged to have one sent to him annually for the rest of his life.)

This community of friends, then, while foremost a gathering of Germans displaced by war and united in this country through personal connections, continued over the years to accrue members based on kindred interests and temperaments. Central to their bond was the force of Dr. Kempner's personality, the devotion of his friends in return for his loyalty, and their commitment to furthering his work. All his life he maintained these strong bonds and continued to attract new friends, bridging gaps of many miles or many years. Robert Boehringer, for example, was thought of as one of the "Neu Dahlem" group, although he never lived in the United States. Dr. Schlayer and Dr. Kempner maintained an active correspondence with him, and their summer trips always included a visit with him, usually at his home in Geneva.

Dr. Kempner maintained his affection for people whom, in a couple of instances, he did not see for as much as fifty years. Around 1980, he came across an article about a young physician whose family name was the same as that of a young girl he had been charmed by in 1918. He wrote the physician, who replied that he was her grandson, and that she was still alive. Dr. Kempner resumed a nostalgic correspondence with her: "Be good and kind to yourself and don't forget the boy who sent you the Faust as a Christmas present 65 years ago." Occasionally he sent her money—"with the provision that you really use it for something nice for yourself and not give it to your grandchildren."

In the summer of 1921, to escape the harsh privations in Germany following World War I, young Walter's mother had sent him out of the country to receive better nourishment and restore his health. She arranged for him to board for a month in Vlieland, Holland, with the family of a Dr. van Terwisga, with whom she had medical connections. Years afterward, Dr. Kempner still remembered that sojourn with warmth and regretted having lost contact with these kind people who had welcomed him into their household. He enlisted the help of the resourceful Helen Mertens to track the family down. To his delight, she located the van Terwisgas' son Piet, with whom Dr. Kempner entered into a warm correspondence and friendship after a lapse of decades. On April 26, 1984, Dr. Kempner wrote,

> I had talked with my friends about your parents and you many times, praising how nice you all were and how many nice things you did for me and to me while I was your guest for at least 5 weeks in Vlieland in the year 1921. I had studied one semester of medicine at this time and was 18 years old. You were age 10 and your worst sin was that you often rushed into the garden without putting on any shoes.
>
> I should appreciate it very much if you would tell me sometime which ages your parents reached and whether they had any annoyances or difficulties during the German occupation.
>
> I am sending you a few of my medical papers which might interest you since you have specialized yourself in internal medicine.
>
> I am also enclosing a check [for 5500 Dutch guilder, or approximately $3000] with which I wish you would get for each of your 11 grandchildren something which might be useful or pleasant.

A friend who entered Dr. Kempner's life in his last years was Katharina Mommsen (born September 18, 1926). She and Dr. Kempner first met at Dr. Schlayer's eighty-eighth birthday party, which Dr. Kempner hosted at his Virginia Avenue house on December 18, 1988. A native of Berlin, Dr. Mommsen was a well-known Goethe scholar, teaching at Stanford University. She had come to Chapel Hill the previous year for a meeting of the German Society, at which time she arranged, through her fellow Germanist Hans Stefan Schultz, to meet Dr. Schlayer. Dr. Mommsen had admired her poetry profoundly. The Schultzes invited her and Dr. Schlayer to tea at their house at 1500 Alabama Avenue, the two women found each other thoroughly congenial, and Dr. Mommsen came from California to visit on several subsequent occasions. She and Dr. Kempner forged an immediate bond through their interest in Goethe, and during her visits to Durham over the years they enjoyed perusing his collection of first editions of Goethe's work.

Since Dr. Kempner lived to the age of 94, he progressively lost many of his friends, yet they continued to figure constantly in his conversation and his life. He took pleasure in recounting stories about departed friends, making them come alive again and keeping them present for himself and us. This attitude

contrasted starkly with my own experience. When I was six years old, my
grandfather died, whereupon my grandmother took to her bed for what I remember as being several weeks. When she finally emerged, she wore black
from then on, and neither she nor anyone else in my family ever mentioned
my grandfather again. I found this bewildering and disturbing. As Goethe says,
in *Egmont*, "*Die Menschen sind nicht nur zusammen, wenn sie beisamen sind, auch
der Enfernte, der Abgeschiedene lebt uns.*" [People are together not only when they
are with each other, but also the distant one, the departed one, lives in us.]

# Development of the Rice Diet

In 1939, while discussing with a group of medical students how the kidney functions as an organ of metabolism as well as excretion, Dr. Kempner suggested that one pathway to kidney failure was through metabolic dysfunction. He explained his hypothesis: The kidneys help break down amino and keto acids derived from protein and fat into useful, or neutral, substances. Normally, these end products either are excreted in urine or circulate harmlessly—even helpfully. However, if blood supply to the kidneys is reduced—by tumor, infection, heart failure or cardiovascular disease—the oxygen-deprived kidney cells may behave abnormally, either producing breakdown products not ordinarily present in the human body or retaining normal substances in abnormal amounts. This throws off the body's acid-base balance; it can also lead to damaged heart and blood vessels, and further damage to the kidneys. The most direct way to break this vicious circle and give the kidneys an opportunity to heal, Dr. Kempner postulated, would be first to decrease their work by radically reducing the amount of fat and protein to be processed, and, second, to increase blood flow—hence oxygen—to the kidneys. He further suggested that, in many cases, both these objectives might be accomplished simply by sharply restricting protein and fat in the patient's diet and virtually eliminating sodium, which impedes blood flow by constricting blood vessels and retaining fluids in body tissue.

One of the students asked why he did not test his theories on patients. Dr. Kempner decided to accept the student's challenge and began applying a diet of rice and fruit to a few patients hospitalized with kidney disease in Duke Hospital's public wards. These patients typically stayed in the hospital for one to four weeks at a time. They were for the most part severely ill, many of them with advanced edema that was already being treated with a protein- and sodium-restricted diet. Dr. Kempner radically reduced further the levels of protein and salt, but because of the patients' precarious condition he proceeded cautiously, modifying the diet as each patient's status required. To the basic rice and fruit he would add some potato, vegetables, a bit of dry toast, and even salt. Among both the terminally and the less seriously ill patients, some of whom were semi-ambulatory, the rice diet's strict reduction of fat, protein, and salt produced dramatic results. After one or more weeks on the diet, edema and uremia (the accumulation of abnormal substances in the blood in kidney failure) decreased, their blood pressure fell significantly, and heart failure disappeared. These initial results strongly reinforced Dr. Kempner's conviction that kidney disease was essentially a matter of metabolic dysfunction. As he refined and applied this treatment that arose rather casually from his discussion with students, his hypothesis would be dramatically confirmed. Moreover, it soon became evident that his diet was effective in patients with hypertension and heart disease unrelated to kidney dysfunction. As Pasteur said, chance favors the prepared mind.

As Dr. Kempner developed it, the rice diet provided about 2000 calories per day, over 95% of which were derived from carbohydrates. Typically, a day's fare consisted of a small bowl of plain rice with a serving of fresh fruit for breakfast, and for lunch and supper a larger serving of rice and two servings of fruit. Fruit juice, served at all three meals, was preferred to water because it was alkaline and compensated for the acidosis present in many kidney patients. The calorie content was adjusted according to whether weight loss or gain was desirable. The daily diet comprised 4–5 percent protein, derived almost entirely from rice, 2–3 percent fat, and the rest carbohydrate. Sodium content was 150 milligrams or less and chloride was 200 milligrams or less. Fluid was restricted to a pint and a half daily, to prevent water intoxication, or dilution of electrolytes. (Contrast this to the "normal" American diet of today, which contains 10–25 percent protein, 20–35 percent fat, 40–60 percent carbohydrates, 7000 milligrams of chloride, and 4000 milligrams of sodium.)

Dr. Kempner was initially able to enforce the rigor necessary to the diet's success because all subjects were hospitalized; their diet was entirely controlled by the medical staff, and the duration of the treatment was relatively short. Physiological responses could be closely monitored. (When the diets were ordered from the hospital kitchen, however, some of the medical staff were horrified and told the patients not to comply. Some may even have smuggled in prohibited food.) Dr. Kempner, usually accompanied by his residents, made daily rounds on his patients, beginning at six thirty in the morning. He obtained measurements of the patients' blood pressure and weight; their blood was checked frequently to measure the concentrations of hemoglobin, nonprotein nitrogen, total protein, chloride, calcium, and phosphorus. Their urine was checked for protein and chloride. He measured kidney function by intravenously injecting phenolsulfonphthalein (PSP) and then measuring the amount excreted in the urine. He also had patients' cholesterol levels measured at a time when scarcely any medical authorities thought there was any connection between cholesterol and disease, or that diet could affect cholesterol levels. After a time, encouraged by the good results achieved in the hospital, Dr.

Kempner pressed the patients to continue the regime as closely as possible after discharge, and to return frequently so that he could monitor their progress.

The results were dramatic. Patients' accumulation of excess fluid (edema) was substantially reduced. One patient lost 63 pounds in 16 days. Patients with heart failure noted great improvement in breathing. A pair of chest x-rays from one particular patient, taken at entry and after treatment with the rice diet, startled Dr. Kempner. Thinking that x-rays from two different patients must have been mixed up, he rushed to the radiology department and asked, "Are these films from the same patient?" Without question, the radiologist assured him, explaining that heart and lung images are as individual as fingerprints. The image clearly showed, much to everyone's surprise and contrary to all previous observations, that the patient's disease-enlarged heart had indeed become smaller. After this stunning revelation, Dr. Kempner ordered sequential electrocardiograms (EKGs) and chest x-rays on all his patients, to see whether this finding would be duplicated. In most cases, the same positive results were obtained. The striking improvement found in treated ward patients soon won over the initially skeptical medical students and interns. As a later class of medical students sang in one of their annual skits, "Isn't it amazin' what you can do with rice and raisins?" Dr. Kempner, if the truth be told, was as surprised as the students. He later recalled,

> [W]e expected that the rice regime, at best, might prevent the usual progressive course of the disease ... However, the chest films and electrocardiograms show that, even in chronic nephritis and hypertensive vascular disease, the rice diet may lead to such an improvement of the heart that it may become normal in size and [the abnormalities in the electrocardiogram may disappear]. Since we did not anticipate these findings, it is only recently that chest films and electrocardiograms of every patient have been repeated after treatment. (*W Kempner 1945a p 11*)

The radical diet was not without pitfalls. On the one hand, even small deviations from the diet could spoil its effect; on the other hand, strict adherence occasionally led to chemical imbalance, particularly when the patient lost excessive sodium or was taking drugs prescribed for some other condition. Several factors might lead to sodium loss: the dysfunctional kidney itself, or diarrhea and vomiting, or even excessive sweating. Among patients with significant kidney disease, fifty-five percent showed major disturbances in serum electrolytes, either initially or within two to three months on the rice diet, leading to modifications in the regimen. For this reason, continued and frequent followup of patients was essential. Ninety-five percent of patients without kidney impairment, however, tolerated the diet well, and some were kept on the basic diet without alteration for many months. (*Peschel & Lohmann Peschel 1952, 1953*)

Dr. Kempner did not consider his radically restricted diet a permanent solution to kidney disease, simply an emergency response to slow or halt kidney deterioration until other, less extreme therapies could be found. At the same time that he began treating his first patients with the rice diet, he and Dr. Schlayer were already searching for simpler treatments, such as a kidney extract that might compensate for the diseased kidney's deficiencies. To this end, Dr. Schlayer had alerted a number of local farmers to notify her when they were ready to slaughter a pig. She would drive out to the farm to retrieve the fresh kidneys and, keeping them in as physiological condition as possible, rush them to the laboratory. The doctors' efforts were not rewarded. Dr. Kempner later [November 6, 1945] wrote to a patient who had inquired about a possible drug treatment,

> Dr. Schlayer here [and I] have tried to extract such "hypotensive," "neutralizing" substances from animal kidneys, but there are still so many technical difficulties in getting these substances in sufficient concentration without toxic by-products that I am afraid that for the time being, patients with hypertension must go the longer and harder way that means they must try to prevent the formation in the body of hypertensive substances. Whenever "hypotensive," "neutralizing" substances can be supplied in sufficient quantity, the patients with hypertension will have a good time again and can enjoy eating and drinking as much as they like.

On September 17, 1942, a 33-year-old woman was admitted to the hospital with terminal chronic nephritis. In addition to her kidney disease she had an enlarged heart, and she was losing her eyesight from retinal hemorrhage and papilledema (swelling of the optic nerve as it enters the eye). Her blood pressure was 190/120. Dr. Kempner placed her on a 1500-calorie, low-sodium, low-protein diet with two quarts of fluids. When she failed to improve after eleven days, Kempner increased the rigor of the diet: nothing but rice, fruit, and one quart of fruit juices. After six days of the stricter treatment, although her blood pressure was unchanged, she felt better and wanted to return home. Dr. Kempner, familiar with the effects of the diet as a short-term treatment for critically ill patients, felt safe in letting her go for a short while, with strict instructions to keep to the diet and return for a checkup in two weeks.

Dr. Kempner's English at this time was still strongly accented (he retained a pronounced German accent all his life), and the patient was a country woman with limited exposure to speech different from her own. Perhaps for that reason she misunderstood the doctor's instructions. Eat rice she did, faithfully and well, but she did not return to the clinic until *two months* later. Dr. Kempner was astonished by what had happened: although her kidney disease was still present, her blood pressure was down to 124/84, her eyesight was normal, and she felt fine. Dr. Kempner instructed her to continue the strict diet at home for another couple of months; again the results were dramatic and positive. With each subsequent checkup he allowed small additions to the diet, without disturbing the good results. After two years of following a liberally modified rice diet, the patient felt "young and strong," resumed a normal workload without fatigue, and had married. Her case was the first to demonstrate that—with the patient's full cooperation—a rigidly restrictive diet could be maintained at home over a significant period of time, that its effectiveness was greatly increased with time, and that the prolonged restriction did no harm to the patient—on the contrary.

Dr. Kempner's radical work was opening the door to a whole new category in the etiology of disease. Only a generation before, when his parents were conducting research, evidence of bacterial and viral origins of disease had still not entirely erased the centuries-old belief that those diseases were caused by "humors" or "miasmas." Researchers were just beginning to understand that diseases like scurvy, beri-beri or pellagra were due to nutritional *deficiency* and, as such, could be cured by vitamin supplements. Now Dr. Kempner's findings indicated that some patients suffered from what might be called diseases of nutritional *excess*. Diseases assumed to be the normal accompaniment of old age, the so-called degenerative diseases, were exacerbated by an excess of protein, sodium, and fat, and—as Dr. Kempner was dramatically demonstrating—could be effectively treated by limiting these dietary components. He wrote:

> Until a few years ago, heart diseases, diabetes mellitus, high blood pressure, obesity, and kidney diseases were not grouped together nor thought to have any common factor. Too many of the factors causing them were unknown. However, there is increasing evidence that these diseases, too, might often have something to do with "external agents," such as some component or components of food, which may act as poisons, not to all but to certain people who are unable to "handle" them. (*WKF Bulletin 1972 p 26*)

Salt restriction as a treatment of hypertension had been tried early in the century, but its effectiveness was limited, in Dr. Kempner's opinion, because the restriction was not drastic enough. As he explained,

Any patient who has suffered from poison ivy knows that it might not help him enough if instead of touching 100 poison ivy leaves he touches only ten or twenty.... With this in mind, it should be possible to understand that in certain diseases ... a decrease from 10 grams to 2 grams [of salt] may be virtually ineffective, and that nevertheless significant changes might occur if the daily salt intake were decreased from 2 grams to 0.3 grams or below. (*W Kempner 1954a p 72*)

As Dr. Kempner was the first to admit, the basic rice diet was monotonous, and many patients had difficulty sticking to it. He and his staff made every effort to make it as agreeable as possible within the necessary limitations. "The palatability of rice," he wrote,

depends to some extent upon the way in which it is cooked. Patients, of course, vary in their tastes; some prefer it dry, each grain standing apart, while others prefer it rather wet.... a little ingenuity in the use of sugar, sliced and preserved fruits, and so forth, will be rewarded. Some patients who object to the sweet taste find the use of lemon juice helpful. Most patients accustom themselves to the rice diet, and some even like it. (*W Kempner 1945a p 62*)

After beginning with the basic diet, patients who showed satisfactory improvement were allowed some modifications, in the form of vegetables and even including small amounts of lean beef, chicken, fish, or eggs, all prepared without salt or fat. The additions usually came at the patient's insistence. Dr. Kempner wrote,

It must be borne in mind, however, that even these slight modifications change the character of the diet and may spoil the entire effect. Where a critical condition of kidney, heart, or retina exists, any compromise may be too much, and the patient may have to pay for the few exceptions made with a reappearance of all the signs and symptoms of the disease. In such cases, the strict diet should be continued indefinitely, just as liver is continued in pernicious anemia* and insulin in diabetes. (*W Kempner 1945a p 63*)

Eleven years later, longer-term data encouraged Dr. Kempner to modify this opinion somewhat:

---

* Initially, the only effective treatment for pernicious anemia was one pound of raw liver consumed daily. When patients complained about the rice diet, Dr. Kempner could point out, quite justly, that it was, at least, far better than the liver treatment.

When treatment with the rice diet was started in 1939, it was thought that extreme dietary restriction would have to be continued indefinitely to compensate for the underlying renal metabolic dysfunction. At present, we have quite a few patients who have been able to resume a salt-poor, fat-poor diet and some who, after an adequate period of intensive treatment, first with strict and then with modified rice diet, have been able to tolerate a general diet without recurrence of vascular disease. (*Newborg & Kempner 1955 p 45*)

When he began using the rice diet, Dr. Kempner was concerned that the very low protein intake might lead to deficiencies of plasma proteins or hemoglobin. He was willing to take those risks, however, because he figured they could be corrected after the imminent dangers of cardiac or kidney failure or of blindness had been overcome. Fortunately periodic blood tests indicated that both plasma proteins and hemoglobin were well maintained on the rice diet. In fact, rice was an excellent choice in all respects as a basis for the diet, because it contains all the essential amino acids and its protein, though small in quantity, is used with great efficiency by the body. As Dr. Kempner pointed out,

[R]ice protein cannot be indiscriminately replaced by other protein. Proteins differ from each other in regard both to the type and the relative proportion of the various amino acids of which they are composed. They also differ in regard to the rate and degree of assimilation; 30 gm. of a protein of which 88% is assimilated may be preferable to 50 gm. of a protein of which only 40% is assimilated. (*W Kempner 1949b p 824*)

The once standard recommendation that 50 grams of protein per day were needed to cover the body's "wear and tear" was based on data derived from patients on a complete fast, whose bodies must consume their own protein as a source of calories. The rice diet might be considered a "protein fast." However, the high carbohydrate content meets the body's energy requirements. Our studies showed that 20 grams of protein from rice were sufficient to prevent any loss of protein from the body. (*W Kempner 1945a; Peschel & Lohmann Peschel 1950*) Consequently, this diet can, with oversight, be carried out indefinitely.

Physicians treating patients with kidney disease gradually accepted Dr. Kempner's teaching that protein intake should be restricted, at least for patients with advanced disease. Over time, some doctors (unfortunately, only a few) saw the wisdom of conserving kidney function by limiting protein intake from the very onset of kidney disease, and they understood that such restriction might be helpful in hypertensive vascular disease and arteriosclerosis where kidney involvement often develops. However, of the major elements of Dr. Kempner's diet program, protein restriction found the least acceptance among both physicians and the public. There is a strongly ingrained societal assumption that animal protein is needed for strength, but powerful animals such as horses and cattle get their strength from grain and grasses; they do not eat meat. The increased popularity of vegetarianism in recent years has shown that health is certainly not impaired, and may be helped, by restricting intake of animal protein. Moreover, in terms of sustainable planetary resources, obtaining protein directly from plants is vastly more efficient than using plants to raise animals which we consume for protein.

Dr. Frederic Hanes, as chairman of the Department of Medicine, watched the progress of his protégé's investigations with keen interest. He noted that the ward patients did very well while they were in the hospital under the restricted diet, but often relapsed at home. Because the department's private patients were typically more prosperous than the ward patients, Dr. Hanes believed they would be able both to arrange longer stays and, not incidentally, to pay. In late 1942 or early 1943, he asked his medical staff and the department business manager to refer some of the hypertensive patients and those with heart or kidney disease to Dr. Kempner. This arrangement, a *de facto* expansion of Dr. Kempner's research and teaching position to include private clinical practice, stirred resentment in the department business office and among many physicians on the Duke medical staff. According to Dr. David Smith, interim chairman of medicine following Dr. Hanes's death in 1946, "They cooperated by referring hospital employees and members of the ministry and their families, whom they would not have charged anyway." (*Wagner et al 1978*) Of thirty-six patients referred by the staff in 1943, the business office sent only fifteen to Dr. Kempner, most of whom were moribund and beyond treatment. Dr. Hanes himself referred three, the Duke student health service referred six, and a few doctors at Duke and in Durham sent an additional twelve patients, also in late stages.

When Dr. Hanes saw that his staff would not voluntarily give up paying patients to Dr. Kempner, he authorized him to recruit his own patients. Dr. Kempner was initially not enthusiastic; he told Dr. Hanes that he had no wish to take on the task of persuading them to go on—and stay on—the rigorous diet. Patients confined to their beds in the public wards were, needless to say, easier to monitor and safer from temptation. Dr. Hanes responded that if Dr. Kempner would see to the medical treatment he, Hanes, would "do the talking" himself.

So Dr. Kempner began seeing patients in the private diagnostic clinic and admitting a number of them to the hospital for extended treatment. With his own patient base, Dr. Kempner acquired from among the house officers a rotating staff assistant, who took initial histories and performed physical examinations on patients at entry. He also acquired a volunteer, who took blood pressures, monitored diets, and provided essential encouragement for the patients.

One day Dr. Hanes received a call from a doctor in Philadelphia, phoning on behalf of one of his patients then in Duke Hospital on the rice diet. The patient had phoned her doctor complaining bitterly of headaches and asked him to intercede to obtain some medication. Dr. Hanes relayed the doctor's message to Dr. Kempner, who duly took the woman a pill but, as he handed it to her, he said, "If you like me, you won't take this." In a few days the headaches had disappeared and did not recur. The patient, reporting her recovery to Dr. Kempner, proudly opened the drawer of her night table and showed him the accumulated pills: she had not taken them after all. Dr. Kempner, reassured that his powers of persuasion were quite adequate to the task, decided that, from then on, he could "do the talking" to the patients himself.

When patients applied for treatment, Dr. Kempner reviewed their initial histories and focused on the most salient points; he then examined every patient himself, listening to the heart, palpating the abdomen, examining the eyegrounds (retina), and checking any abnormal findings noted in the admitting examination. The extensive battery of entry tests initially required up to ten days to complete because of the time-consuming kidney tests and problems in scheduling some of the procedures. As the procedures became more standardized and streamlined, results became available in only two or three days. Dr. Kempner personally summarized the findings and recommendations to each patient. He would often spend an hour trying to persuade a patient of the seriousness of his condition, the relative inconsequence of social and business obligations, and the necessity of submitting to prolonged treatment.

# Results

As Dr. Kempner had pointed out to the medical students, his research had strongly indicated that a radical reduction of sodium, protein, and fat could halt or at least slow the disease process in patients with damaged kidneys. He had not imagined that, also in hypertensive patients with no evidence of kidney disease, the rice diet could actually reduce blood pressure, reverse heart failure, heal retinopathy, and, most astonishingly, significantly shrink disease-enlarged hearts. But remarkable results were achieved in some of his early patients on the wards. As the successes mounted, Dr. Kempner broadened his research to include patients admitted for valvular and coronary heart disease, whose response confirmed the rice diet to be a consistently successful intervention in a range of disorders—although in some stubborn cases only when it was continued over years.

Finally Dr. Hanes persuaded Dr. Kempner that it was time to make his discoveries more widely known. On May 8, 1944, at a meeting of the North Carolina Medical Society in Pinehurst, North Carolina, Dr. Kempner presented the findings publicly for the first time. He opened his talk with disarming candor:

> It is a greater pleasure to talk for fifteen minutes about the treatment of kidney disease and hypertensive vascular disease with the rice diet than to eat this diet three times daily for fifteen days, or fifteen weeks, or fifteen months. Let me start with a number of unpleasant facts: (1) This is a monotonous diet and it does not taste good. It can never become popular. (2) One has to eat it for quite a while before its full effect becomes apparent. (3) The patients should be in the hospital until they are "regulated" on the diet, and constant checks on their blood and urine chemistry should be made. (4) The diet becomes worthless if it is modified by so-called "small" or "minimal" additions according to the patient's own taste....
>
> There is only one excuse for such a therapy: it helps, and if there is a choice between an unpleasant diet on the one side and cardiac failure, uremia, encephalopathy, or blindness on the other side, I think the diet is the lesser evil. (*W Kempner 1944c p 273*)

He accompanied his presentation with a profusion of charts, x-ray and eyeground photographs, and electrocardiographic (EKG) readouts—scrupulously doc-

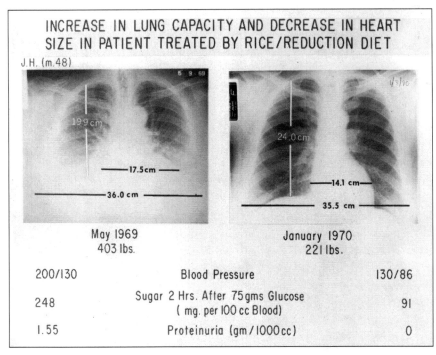

INCREASE IN LUNG CAPACITY AND DECREASE IN HEART SIZE IN PATIENT TREATED BY RICE/REDUCTION DIET

J.H. (m.48)

| May 1969 403 lbs. | | January 1970 221 lbs. |
|---|---|---|
| 200/130 | Blood Pressure | 130/86 |
| 248 | Sugar 2 Hrs. After 75 gms Glucose ( mg. per 100 cc Blood) | 91 |
| 1.55 | Proteinuria (gm / 1000 cc) | 0 |

Figure 33. Patient with obesity, hypertensive vascular disease and diabetes showed return to normal heart and lung size after 8 months on rice diet.

umenting not only the remarkable results of treatment but also the careful monitoring needed to ensure both patients' safety in the course of radical dietary change and their adherence to the regime.

Six weeks after the North Carolina meeting, in June 1944, Dr. Kempner presented his findings in a poster exhibit and an address at the annual meeting of the American Medical Association in Chicago. His audience was stunned by his presentation and the irrefutable evidence of his documentation. Some physicians, however, seeing the x-ray evidence of reduction in heart size, accused Kempner of fraud, insisting that he must have reversed the dates on the images. Dr. Hanes consoled Dr. Kempner for these attacks on his integrity, urging him not to pay any attention to "those blasted Yankees." Kempner's response was, "If the only way they can explain my results is to call them forgeries, then I must have done something rather remarkable!"

The AMA customarily published papers presented at its national meetings; however, it withheld its invitation to publish Dr. Kempner's presentation, apparently because of the lively controversy and publicity surrounding it. On

June 26, Kempner wrote to Dr. Morris Fishbein, editor of the Journal of the American Medical Association:

> Could you let me know when it is likely to be decided whether or not the paper "Treatment of Kidney Disease and Hypertensive Vascular Disease with Rice Diet" which I read at the AMA Symposium on hypertension, June 15th, will be published in the JAMA.

Two months later, responding to a query from Dr. Hanes, Kempner wrote:

> The AMA has refused to print the Chicago talk, I suppose on the suggestion of the chairman of the section, the gentleman from Cleveland with the white belt and shoes whose face you did not like. The reason given by Dr. Fishbein, that no comparison with "subminimal diets" had been made, is not very convincing since I think the main question is not whether any other diet may have the same effect, but whether this diet can actually produce such changes in blood pressure, heart, eye, etc. as we were able to show.
>
> Since I did not receive Dr. Fishbein's letter until a few days ago, the paper was only sent on August 1st to the Archives of Internal Medicine. I hope their answer will be different from that of the AMA, but I am afraid this rice treatment has stirred up a good deal of controversy, both pro and contra, which is not entirely concerned with the objective findings.

On August 21, 1944, Dr. Kempner wrote again to Hanes saying he had not heard from the Archives and adding,

> I think your suggestion to publish it in the North Carolina Journal is very good. Do you think they could publish a lot of pictures?

The North Carolina Medical Journal agreed to publish the long paper, complete with illustrations—a major undertaking. The assistant editor wrote [October 19, 1944], "As to the beautiful hearts and charts and eyes, we shall be delighted to publish all you want—but unfortunately at Duke's expense. I regret that we cannot make an exception to this rule, even in your case."* On November 17: "Start getting your paper ready as quickly as possible, for the world and I are both waiting with baited [sic] breath for the final, complete and authoritative word on the Kempner regime." This unprecedentedly (for the Journal) voluminous paper had a somewhat difficult birth, generating a constant but congenial correspondence between the assistant editor and Dr. Kempner.

---

* In fact, it was Dr. Kempner, not Duke, who paid these charges.

Finally, in the February/March 1945 issues, the two-part, 72-page article appeared. (*W Kempner 1945a, 1945b*) In the meantime, the study sample had grown from 150 to 213 patients. The article included over 70 illustrations—tables, charts, electrocardiograms, chest x-rays, and eyeground photographs—and case histories of ten patients. The tremendous amount of painstaking, highly technical work required for the Duke Department of Medical Art and Illustration to produce the final publication was carried out by Dr. Clotilde Schlayer, at that time Dr. Kempner's only associate. In summary, these were the results presented:

*Blood pressure*: Of 192 patients with hypertension from primary kidney disease or hypertensive vascular disease, many were already gravely ill or moribund on arrival, and unable to be effectively treated by the diet. Of these, 25 died. In the surviving 167, 60 showed no significant improvement in blood pressure (average decrease from 196/120 to 180/114 after an average of 39 days on the diet); 107 showed significant improvement (average decrease from 200/122 to 149/96 after an average of 62 days on the diet).

*Heart size*: Before-and-after heart measurements were available for 72 patients. Of these, six patients showed an increase in heart size (average 3.2%) and 66 showed a decrease (average of 13.3%).

*Cholesterol*: Serum cholesterol was measured, both before and after treatment, in 82 patients on the rice diet for an average of 91 days. Nine showed increased cholesterol; the remaining 73 showed a decrease, from an average of 266 to an average 183 mg/dL of serum. (Dr. Kempner at that time considered normal to be between 120 and 220 mg/dL.)

*Retinopathy*: Of 33 patients with advanced vascular retinal changes (papilledema, hemorrhages, or exudates), who followed the diet for at least eight weeks, one patient's retinopathy worsened; in 11, the progress of the retinopathy was halted and the papilledema, hemorrhages, and exudates partially cleared up; in the remaining 21, the retinopathy improved greatly or cleared completely.

In addition to these findings, the paper described several other responses to the treatment which, because they were more subjective and episodic, were not quantified:

> A great number of patients on the rice diet have experienced marked relief from giddiness, headache, mental sluggishness and depression, and easy fatiguability. Such *subjective* improvement has not been accepted as evidence of successful therapy; only *objective* results, such as the loss of edema and changes in the urine and blood chemistry findings, in blood pressure, eyegrounds, heart size, and electrocardiograms, have been used to determine the effects of the treatment. (*W Kempner 1945a p 63*)

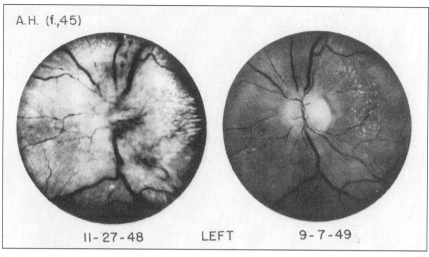

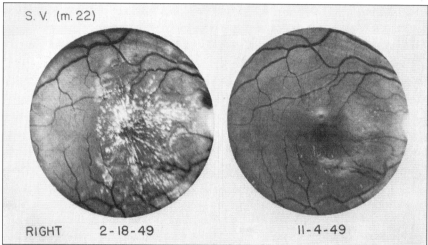

Figures 34 & 35. The eyeground, or back of the eyeball, is the only place where blood vessels are noninvasively visible and thus provide valuable information on the state of vascular health. The upper set of before-and-after eyeground photos shows a case of advanced papilledema in a hypertensive patient. At left, the optic nerve is completely obscured by swelling, hemorrhage from the engorged veins, and exudates (white area). The photo at right shows only minimal remaining exudates and a normal optic nerve. The lower set is from a patient with chronic nephritis, showing extensive exudation or leakage of fluid from the blood vessels in the macula. Nine months later, the macula is almost entirely clear.

It may be useful at this point to examine more closely the nature of the major diseases successfully treated by Dr. Kempner and to give some specifics on the changes brought about by the rice diet.

## Hypertension, Benign and Malignant

*Benign, or essential, hypertension* denotes high blood pressure of unknown cause, often persisting for many years and, at least initially, unaccompanied by complications in the heart, kidneys, or eyegrounds. Because the condition can persist for long periods without overt symptoms—hence the designation "benign"—it has most often been left untreated. But Dr. Kempner believed that hypertension over time invariably leads to more overt, life-threatening conditions, and he always stressed that it should, and could, be treated whenever it was detected and before the more incapacitating complications of the disease have developed (cardiac breakdown, cerebral accidents, loss of vision, and renal insufficiency).

> Old age is considered by most of us a kind of bankruptcy, caused by the accumulation of vascular, cardiac, and renal debts. Accordingly, the arteriosclerotic and hypertensive vascular processes are accepted as results of degenerative disease, an inevitable and almost physiologic accompaniment of advancing years. The reversibility of some of these processes in many of my older patients proves, however, that this attitude of resignation is today no longer necessary. (*W Kempner 1954a p 85*)

He continually emphasized the importance of aggressive early treatment of even mild elevations of blood pressure, rather than the all too common acceptance of this "normal" accompaniment of aging.

> The systolic blood pressure of a person of seventy-five, just as well as that of a person of thirty, should be below 130, the diastolic below 90. A consoling remark such as, "A blood pressure of 175/110 is good enough at this age," is an unwarranted admission of defeat and should not be substituted for active treatment. It denotes an attitude reminiscent of the days when similar excuses were given with regard to the "diseases of early infancy," instead of treating specific diseases by specific methods. (*W Kempner 1954a p 85*)

In *malignant hypertension*, which may arise spontaneously or develop in patients with benign hypertension, the diastolic blood pressure is extremely high and is accompanied by papilledema, or swelling of the optic nerve. When Dr. Kempner initiated the rice diet treatment, a diagnosis of malignant hypertension was considered a death sentence, as most patients died within three to six months. There was an early and dramatic demonstration that malignant hypertension was in fact both treatable and reversible: a moderately obese 24-year-old woman was admitted to the hospital in November 1944 with severe headaches, steadily decreasing vision, enlarged heart, and blood pressure of 233/157. After four months on the rice diet, her heart size had decreased from 16.6 to a normal 12.9 centimeters, her headaches had disappeared, her vision was greatly improved, and her blood pressure was 121/87. She continued to follow a modified rice diet at home and returned for periodic checkups for about five years, during which time, despite her less than perfect adherence to the diet, she maintained pretty good health. She was still alive and in functioning health nine years later.

Many patients did not stay the prescribed length of time, and there was little one could do except try to convince them their decision was unwise. When a 45-year-old man came to Dr. Kempner from New York in October 1947, he had had hypertension for at least five years, and it was now malignant, with marked papilledema in both eyes and blood pressure of 210/140; he also suffered from asthma. But his response to the rice diet was excellent. After only one week his blood pressure had dropped to 160/118, and after nine weeks it was 100/74. He had developed diarrhea, however, which weakened him, and his electrolytes went badly out of balance. Although he was urged to stay, he insisted on returning home and left with a diet to which some vegetables had been added.

At home his condition continued to deteriorate; he was very weak and his blood pressure was down. In a conference call with Dr. Kempner, his doctor insisted on hospital admission in New York for intravenous saline. Dr. Kempner's suggestion was to give him some toast and get him on the plane for Durham right away. The patient's wife, who had great confidence in Dr. Kempner after the dramatic results of her husband's first visit, overrode the New York physician's opinion and agreed to Dr. Kempner's plan, and the patient was admitted at Duke Hospital. By this time his standing blood pressure was 60/30, and his chloride levels were critically low. For the first week, his rice diet was supplemented with nine slices of regular toast daily; the next week, six slices of toast, four ounces of chicken, two tomatoes, and two potatoes daily; toast was then discontinued but the chicken and vegetables were continued. After eight to ten days he felt well and could walk around, and in the third week he was over the incident. Other than a small amount of cortisone administered twice shortly after admission, he received no other medication. It was later ascertained, on a subsequent admission, that the dangerous drop in his chloride levels was due primarily to prolonged asthma attacks in which the patient expectorated large amounts of sputum. (*W Kempner 1949a*)

The patient kept in contact with Dr. Kempner over the next years, sending us serum samples for electrolyte determinations as well as urine specimens. We altered his diet from time to time accordingly. In the fall of 1955, he spent three and a half weeks in Durham for treatment, and a few days on four subsequent occasions for re-examination and adjustment of treatment, which in his case was complicated by the asthma. At times he received steroids for his asthma. Dr. Kempner continued to exhort him, as he did all his patients, to make his health his top priority. In June 1957, following one of his visits, Dr. Kempner wrote him,

> It is true you have made remarkable progress during the past ten years. However, your vascular disease is again active and I, therefore, would like to repeat what I have told you on various occasions, that you should plan to spend some time here under our supervision so that the optimal regime can be worked out for you. I realize the inconveniences and difficulties involved but since this is an insidious disease, you should not be content with your present state of health.

In 1961 examination by Dr. Kempner showed that he was holding his own except for increased blood pressure, for which he again elected not to stay for treatment. In January 1963, for reasons that still are not clear, his kidneys gradually shut down. He died in February 1963. In her letter reporting on the final weeks of life his wife wrote to Dr. Kempner, "I feel that I am greatly indebted to you for the 16 years of Gene's life, and I know he would feel the same."

## Nephritis and Nephrosis

*Nephritis* refers to inflammation of the tissues and small vessels of the kidney, so that the glomeruli tubules responsible for clearing waste products from the blood are obstructed or otherwise malfunction. The resulting build-up of waste (uremia) slowly poisons the patient. Nephritis is characterized by the presence of abnormal amounts of red blood cells and protein in the urine and is often accompanied by high blood pressure, heart enlargement, and changes in the eyegrounds.

A 32-year-old farmer's wife with chronic nephritis was admitted in February 1943 in a semi-comatose state, with a blood pressure of 250/174, an enlarged heart, and eyegrounds showing papilledema, hemorrhages, and exudates. She was immediately started on the rice diet, but because of vomiting had to receive some supplementary intravenous nourishment. There was marked uremia in her blood, but after six weeks the uremia cleared, although her kidney function tested at about one-fifth normal. After 52 days she was discharged to continue the diet at home — which she did quite well — and to return for a checkup in five weeks. At that time her blood pressure was 130/102, the papilledema, exudates, and hemorrhages had disappeared, and her eyesight was fully restored. When next seen, six months after her initial workup, she was unfortunately no longer following the diet well, and her blood pressure had risen to 220/160. She became lost to follow-up, and we learned nothing further.

A somewhat better outcome was achieved with another young woman, admitted in April 1943 with chronic nephritis, blood pressure of 246/159, and abnormal eyegrounds. During six weeks in the hospital she responded well to first a strict and then a modified rice diet. After discharge she returned several times for checkups and was found to be doing well. Seven months later, however, she returned to the hospital with diarrhea, loss of appetite, and weakness from gastroenteritis. Her serum sodium was dangerously low and was successfully corrected by adding salt to the diet for a few days. A year after her initial hospital stay, having followed a slightly modified rice diet and without receiving medications, her blood pressure was 116/92, her cholesterol had decreased from 270 to 148, and her eyegrounds had improved. There was still some protein in her urine, but it had decreased from 1.65gm/liter to 0.28 (normal is less than 0.03). She continued to do well for several years, but after five or six years she abandoned the diet and died of cardio-renal failure within a year.

In 1940, Dr. George Minot (1885–1950), a Nobel-winning Harvard hematologist, came by Dr. Kempner's office while on a visit to Duke. I presume this was out of curiosity about the rice program; the two were not acquainted. Their talk turned to whether it was possible for damaged kidneys to regenerate. Still in the earliest stages of his investigations with the rice diet, Dr. Kempner expressed doubt that such an outcome was possible. He was convinced that the manifestations of kidney disease could be controlled, but he doubted that the kidney itself could heal. Dr. Minot replied, "Use your treatment for longer periods of time and you will see the kidney recover." Minot proved to be right. In a group of 76 patients with malignant hypertension who were treated for five years or longer, 79 percent showed an increase in excretion rates (PSP) averaging from 53 to 69 percent. As Dr. Minot had predicted, *duration* of treatment was an important factor. In a paper published five years after Dr. Minot's death, we noted,

> It usually takes at least three to four months of intensive dietary treatment to produce a significant decrease in the heart size and blood pressure.... For improvement in kidney function, at least two to three years are needed. (*Newborg & Kempner 1955 p 45*)

One of the first of Dr. Kempner's cases to confirm the possibility of regenerating severely damaged kidneys was that of an acutely ill 24-year-old woman, five feet three inches tall and weighing 194 pounds, who, in June 1954, came to Dr. Kempner seeking treatment after two weeks of constant nausea. Initial examination showed a blood pressure of 200/140 and virtually no kidney function: her excretion rate of PSP was only 3.5% (a normal rate is 85% or more), and she was uremic. The patient was diagnosed with nephritis and admitted to the hospital to start the rice diet. At first, because of the nausea, she was unable to eat anything and had to be fed puréed rice through a stomach tube, but soon she was able to take the diet orally. Because of her decreased kidney function her electrolyte levels were closely monitored, with small amounts of bread or vegetables added to the rice diet as needed to keep the electrolytes in balance.

By the time she was discharged four months later, her condition had improved greatly in several ways: her blood pressure had been normal for two months, her electrolyte values were normal; the uremia had decreased; her kidney function (as measured by the PSP), while still low, had improved. She weighed 150 pounds—still too much, but a great improvement over 194 pounds. In March 1956, after less than two years on a modified rice diet, the patient came for her seventh check-up visit. Although she had let her salt intake creep up higher than it should have been, her health had continued to improve. She weighed 128 pounds and, best of all, her kidney function had increased to 30 percent. (*WKF Bulletin 1956 p 23*) Our records show that she lived sixteen years after her initial treatment by Dr. Kempner.

*Nephrosis* is a kidney disease characterized by large amounts of protein in the urine, generalized edema, low serum protein and high serum cholesterol. It is usually not accompanied by the high blood pressure or excessive blood nitrogen that characterize chronic nephritis. Nephrosis most frequently occurs in young children, and usually lasts for months up to three years, by which time it has resolved either in healing or kidney failure. As early as 1946, Dr. Kempner had already successfully treated with the rice diet a four-year-old nephrotic child, who made a complete recovery in two years. In 1949 he reported for the first time on the effect of rice diet in a nephrotic patient. (*W Kempner 1949b*)

A 13-year-old girl arrived in June 1948 with massive swelling of her abdomen and chest from fluid retention. In treatment elsewhere, she had already had 11 liters of fluid drained from her abdomen and, separately, a liter of fluid from her chest, but the fluids kept re-accumulating. In the first four months of treatment with rice diet, most of the excess fluid was excreted, and she lost sixty pounds; her cholesterol fell from 540 to 185 mg/dL, and her serum protein and albumin levels improved. Protein excretion in her urine decreased from 10.1 grams to .17 grams (normal less than .03). After leaving the hospital, she kept in touch with us for many years, writing to report happily that, on an almost normal diet, she continued in good health and had borne a child after an uneventful pregnancy—an outcome that could scarcely have been imagined earlier. This patient was one of a number of nephrotic children whom Dr. Kempner treated beginning in 1946, whose recovery confirmed yet another important application of the rice diet and demonstrated that the diet contained sufficient high-class protein to sustain healthy growth.

One of our most memorable nephrotic patients was a very sick five-year-old boy from Tacoma, Washington, who had already been hospitalized repeatedly. On arrival he weighed 51 pounds, of which 20 were fluid. His abdomen had been tapped several times to relieve his acute edema, but the fluid quickly returned; he had received four blood transfusions and some injections of albumin. He was started immediately on the rice diet and stayed on the diet, in Durham, for 31 weeks. (Asked how he was able to follow the diet so much better than many of the adults, he replied, "I guess I'm just used to it.") His edema disappeared; his serum cholesterol decreased from 1,100 to 305 mg/dL; his serum protein increased and his urine protein decreased. At the time he was discharged his diet included unlimited amounts of fruits and vegetables, five ounces of pasta daily, and three ounces of meat per week. (*W Kempner 1954a*) For the next seven years, he spent six or seven weeks annually in Durham for additional treatment. We followed his progress for 40 years, during which he came back five more times. Aside from a trace of protein in the urine and an occasional mildly elevated blood pressure, he remained well. He has married, had two children, and works as a journalist.

Dr. Kempner had an adult patient, 58 years old, who came to him a year after developing nephrosis. After a year on the rice diet, her disease was in remission, and in the next year she gradually discontinued treatment. About three years later, the edema recurred, so she returned and stayed for five months of renewed treatment; again she went into remission. We followed her for several years after this second session and found that, having learned her lesson, she had been able to stick to the diet and was leading an active, evidently healthy life. (*WKF Bulletin 1958 p 25*)

Dr. Eugene Stead, Frederic Hanes's distinguished successor as head of the Department of Medicine, considered this successful treatment of nephrosis one of Dr. Kempner's greatest achievements with the rice diet. "Before Dr. Kempner's work," he declared,

> we believed that a patient with little protein in the blood, who was losing a large amount of protein in the urine, would have died on such a protein intake.... Who in his right mind would have ever thought that rice and fruit could modify vascular disease appreciably? ... Who would have dared to give a more than 90% carbohydrate diet to a diabetic? Every expert knew that cholesterol levels were not

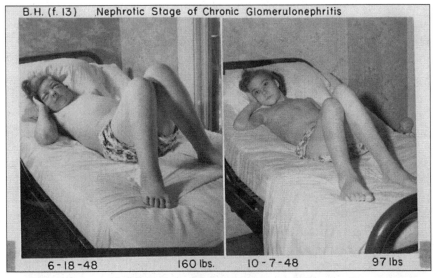

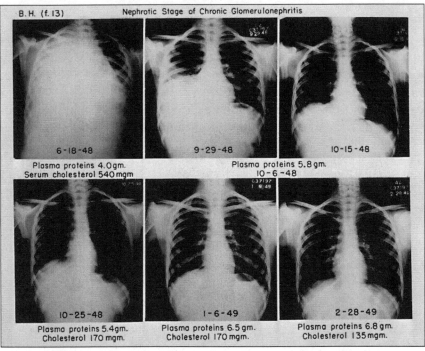

Figures 36 & 37.  Nephrotic patient admitted with extreme edema at age 13,
seen at entry and after four months on rice diet. X-rays show her fluid-filled
chest cavity at entry and progressive improvement over treatment.

influenced by diet. Nevertheless, all these leads have paid off richly. (*WKF Bulletin 1956 p 6*)

## Arteriosclerosis

Arteriosclerosis is a chronic disease that produces hardening, thickening, and loss of elasticity in the arteries, reducing or even halting blood flow. This condition is the basis of coronary artery disease, peripheral vascular disease, and other vascular problems, including stroke.

In *coronary artery disease*, the blood flow in one or more of the coronary arteries (so named because of their vaguely crown shape) normally feeding the heart muscle is reduced or blocked; in the latter case, the blood-deprived muscle tissue served by that artery actually dies, and is replaced by scar tissue, the process known as a myocardial infarction—or, in lay terminology, a heart attack or "coronary." While the heart continues to function in a majority of cases, ten to forty percent of first infarctions are fatal. In less severe blockages, when the heart tissue survives and continues to function despite greater or lesser degrees of damage, there is often associated pain, which we call angina pectoris.

Even after the rice diet's effectiveness in treating heart, eye, and kidney diseases became acknowledged, it was not widely understood that coronary artery disease was responsive to the treatment as well. By 1947, however, Dr. Kempner was successfully treating patients with coronary artery disease, in order "to counteract or to prevent those processes which lead to a decrease in coronary blood flow and to reduce the energy requirements of the myocardium (heart muscle)." (*W Kempner 1954a p 77*) That year he published the case history of a 45-year-old man admitted to the hospital with a myocardial aneurysm following an infarction. His kidney function was normal, his blood pressure was normal, but he was in severe cardiac failure. During 15 weeks on the rice diet he lost 50 pounds; his heart decreased in size from 19.75 to 17.15 centimeters; his edema, shortness of breath, and liver enlargement disappeared; his waist size went from 110 to 83 centimeters. He continued to do well for five years, then suffered a fatal heart attack. Although Dr. Kempner did not conclusively demonstrate (as Dean Ornish would later) the actual reversal of arteriosclerotic lesions in the coronary arteries, we had substantial empirical evidence that this was occurring. It is frustrating to observe, in the twenty-first century, that despite the frequent occurrence of heart failure or stroke in patients being treated for coronary artery disease, the essential role of diet in forestalling these consequences is still widely ignored.

*Peripheral vascular disease*, or impaired blood flow in vessels leading to the legs and lower body, is another manifestation of arteriosclerosis. Symptoms associated with it include impotence and claudication (leg pain on walking).

Many patients have had these problems reversed by strict adherence to the rice diet. This result is due not only to the reduction in dietary fat but also to sodium and protein restriction. The most striking example of improvement that I have witnessed was in a patient who because of claudication could not walk more than three or four steps without pain. After the rice diet treatment, he took three-mile walks with ease.

One of the first patients Dr. Kempner treated with the rice diet, a leading industrialist with hypertension, reported that, along with other symptoms, he suffered from impotence. Dr. Kempner told him that, unfortunately, he doubted that this condition could be relieved. When, months later, the patient returned for a check-up examination, he greeted Dr. Kempner with the words, "You're not much of a physician!" "Why?" asked Dr. Kempner, surprised. "You said I'd never be able to resume a normal sex life, but things haven't been this good since I first married." "Who's the lucky girl?" "My wife!"

Reflecting on this and similar situations, Dr. Kempner said,

> No life of any plant, no animal life, no human life without oxygen. And how many diseases are due to lack of oxygen! 'Lavoisier,'* I have said many times, sitting in front of my fireplace, before using the bellows to revive the fire, and to my patients I said: What you call narcolepsy or stroke, I call insufficient oxygen in the brain. What you call heart attack, I call insufficient oxygen in the heart muscle. What you call impotence, I call insufficient oxygen in the testes and their surroundings. (*WKF Bulletin 1993 p 13*)

## Cholesterol

As early as 1942, Dr. Kempner began measuring his patients' cholesterol levels, although at that time the relation of cholesterol to heart attack and stroke was not recognized, nor was it thought that the level could be influenced in any way. The great majority of Dr. Kempner's patients, however, showed a reduction of cholesterol levels on the rice diet, and in a 1948 paper he made a case for the role of elevated serum cholesterol in the development of vascular disease, stating,

> Hypercholesterolemia, regardless of its primary cause in a given case, is just as significant a metabolic disturbance as persistent hyperglycemia or hyperuricemia and should probably be considered as serious a dis-

---

* Antoine Lavoisier, a French scientist, recognized and named oxygen and hydrogen in 1778.

ease, as far as potential consequences are concerned, as diabetes mellitus and gout. (*W Kempner 1948 p 550*)

In May 1955, Dr. Kempner admitted for treatment a 32-year-old man with a cholesterol level of 504; subcutaneous cholesterol deposits (xanthomas) covered his hands and elbows. After seven months on the diet, his cholesterol had decreased to 289. Two years from commencement of treatment, it was 207, and the xanthomas had disappeared. In an even more striking case, a patient came to Dr. Kempner in 1979 with cholesterol of 1,284 and triglycerides of 9,879! This 52-year-old businessman had an interesting history. In addition to high cholesterol, high blood pressure, for which he was on medication, and untreated diabetes, he suffered from chronic heartburn, which he relieved with milk. For years he had consumed a quart of milk daily; by the time he came to Dr. Kempner his intake had increased to two to four quarts a day. He weighed 272 pounds and had erupting xanthomas (small yellow papules) covering his knees, elbows, arms, and buttocks. When his blood was drawn and sent to several laboratories for routine determinations, the technicians were stunned to see a milky-colored fluid: his blood was so full of fat that some determinations could not be made. They could measure his blood sugar concentration: at 8:30 a.m. (fasting) it was 483mg/100cc; 600 before lunch; 744 in late afternoon. Normal blood sugars are 60 to 100. He was started on the rice diet, supplemented for the first 43 days by insulin. Over three or four weeks, his blood pressure medication was gradually discontinued. At discharge, after 231 days, he was not taking any medication, he had lost 106 pounds, and his blood pressure was normal (114/74), as was his blood sugar. The cholesterol concentration had decreased to 265, and triglycerides to 102; most of the xanthomatous eruptions had disappeared.

While not every case we saw was as impressive as these two, the results achieved with rice diet on patients with high cholesterol were consistently rewarding.

## Diabetes Mellitus

In 1948 Dr. Kempner described the use of the rice diet in treating diabetes mellitus. Because complications of the eyes, kidneys, and heart are commonly associated with diabetes, patients coming to Dr. Kempner for treatment of these conditions often also had diabetes. The idea of submitting these patients to a high-carbohydrate diet was radically contrary to current understanding, because carbohydrates were considered particularly contraindicated in diabetes. The recommended treatment at that time contained less than half the carbohydrate of the rice diet, with approximately three times as much protein, ten times as much fat, and more than 25 times as much sodium. Speaking of his success with the rice diet, Dr. Kempner reported,

> It was expected that in order to maintain the previous blood sugar levels larger amounts of insulin would have to be given. We found instead that in many cases the blood sugar decreased on the rice diet and the insulin dose had to be reduced. (*W Kempner 1948a p 561*)

Dr. Kempner had read of a few advanced cases of diabetes being treated surgically, by removal of the adrenal or pituitary glands. The involvement of the adrenal gland in elevation of blood sugar had already been described by him in his very first published paper on phlorizin diabetes, in 1927. Subsequent observations only strengthened his conviction that there was an important connection:

> The sugar in the blood increases under the influence of adrenalin.... It is often said that high blood sugar is caused by the inefficiency of the pancreas because of too little insulin, but one rarely hears that it is due to a hyperactive adrenal gland producing too much adrenalin. And "thereby hangs a tale": DEPRESSION OF ADRENAL ACTIVITY BY REMOVAL OF SODIUM. (*W Kempner 1993 p 11*)

Dr. Kempner felt that the sodium reduction afforded by the rice diet led to increased insulin sensitivity in diabetic patients. He considered that he was thus able to achieve a reversible inactivation of the adrenal and pituitary glands "in a conservative and unbloody way."

In diabetic patients, the development of retinopathy was considered an irreversible and ominous sign; most patients with a combination of neovascularization (new blood vessel growth), hemorrhages, and exudates became blind within a few years and died within six or seven years. In 1950 a young man came to the clinic with a nine-year history of diabetes. His disease had seemed to be quite well controlled until, six months before coming to us, he noted blurred vision. He could read only large print, and his eyegrounds showed changes characteristic of diabetes: When diabetes damages the retinal arteries, the "detour" of blood around the blockage stimulates formation of new blood vessels; these frail new vessels are subject to rupture, resulting in hemorrhage in the eyes. It is possible to restore normal blood flow; either one or more of the temporary vessels may grow large enough to handle the volume, or the occluded vessel may occasionally heal and reopen. We do not fully understand the mechanisms involved in the latter case, but our eyeground photographs after the rice diet treatment have repeatedly shown restoration of flow in the blocked vessels. After extended treatment with the rice diet, this young man's eyegrounds were virtually clear. By 1955 he could read small print with his left eye, and he was able to resume work until his death twenty years later. Such experience, Dr. Kempner declared,

> leads us to conclude that an attitude of resignation with regard to the prognosis in diabetes mellitus with vascular complications, including diabetic retinopathy, is no longer necessary. The course of the disease can be favorably changed by intensive treatment with the rice diet. (*W Kempner et al 1958 p 371*)

A government official from Melbourne, Australia, wrote Dr. Kempner in January 1966 asking for details on the diet after his diabetic eye disease had begun to interfere with his ability to carry out his duties. Dr. Kempner sent reprints of several research articles to him and to his physicians, and the man started his own rice diet treatment at home in mid-February. Over the next 18 months, with the help of his Australian doctor, a diabetes clinic, and Dr. Kempner's input by mail, he tried to maintain the diet. He succeeded in slowing his disease, but his eyesight continued to deteriorate, and finally he came to Durham. When he arrived in August 1967 he was 52 years old, had had diabetes for over 20 years, and had been on insulin the whole time. He had an elevated blood pressure, kidney damage, and eye damage. After the four months he had initially allotted for treatment, during which he made excellent progress, Dr. Kempner asked him whether he would consider prolonging his stay. The patient replied, "I leave that to your intuition, doctor." He ended up staying seven and a half months, at the end of which his eyesight was sufficiently improved that he was able to resume his job at home, where word of his success must have spread: The 1968 nutrition manual of the Melbourne Hospital includes a copy of the Kempner diet.

From Australia the patient and his doctors stayed in close contact with Dr. Kempner, reporting blood pressure readings, sugar levels, etc. Even at that distance, Dr. Kempner maintained the strict surveillance that he imposed on all his patients: Between April 1968 and October 1969, the patient air-mailed fifty-three urine specimens in small two-ounce containers, so that they could be analyzed to monitor his adherence to the diet, which usually proved to be good. In October 1969 the man returned to Durham for a few days for a check-up; between his return home and his second short six-day visit in March of 1973, he sent another eighty urine specimens. In 1971 or 1972 he began to develop peripheral neuropathy, which gave him considerable trouble walking, but he was improving by the late summer of 1973. In September, busy planning a new building and new developments for his staff, he became ill and was diagnosed with an abscess in the gall bladder. Upon operating, the surgeons found

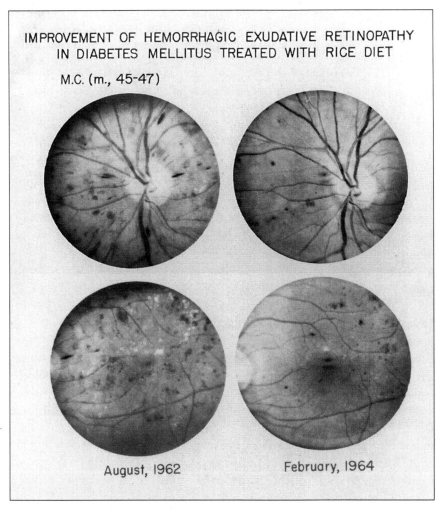

IMPROVEMENT OF HEMORRHAGIC EXUDATIVE RETINOPATHY
IN DIABETES MELLITUS TREATED WITH RICE DIET

M.C. (m., 45-47)

August, 1962            February, 1964

Figure 38. The before-and-after eyeground images at top show decreased
hemorrhage (black spots). The lower images of the same eye, photographed
at a different angle, also show clearing of exudates (white spots).

stones in the gall bladder and in the common duct, and the surgery, which
was to have been minor and short, instead lasted two hours. The patient failed
to recover. On October 22, his wife wrote to tell Dr. Kempner,

> I would like you to know that in the past few weeks he had begun to
> plan his retirement with a real sense of enjoyment and that first he
> planned to come to Durham as he had promised. Then he looked for-

ward to having time to enjoy his family and friends. Alan and I were both grateful for the eight wonderful years you gave us, bonus years in which he saw our three children married ...

A 63-year-old woman was admitted in 1954 with a five-year history of diabetes. She was on a sweet-restricted diet, and for a year and a half had been taking 90 units of insulin daily. After a few weeks on the rice diet, her blood sugar decreased markedly and the insulin was reduced. After four months, her insulin dose was only 20 units and her sugar was normal. Instead of returning home the patient asked if she could stay longer, with the goal of discontinuing insulin altogether. Five months after admission, insulin was discontinued and her blood sugar remained satisfactory. In this case, weight loss was certainly not a factor; her weight was 114 pounds on admission and 109 pounds at discharge. She was followed in our clinic until 1963 and continued to do well. We later learned from her husband that she died in 1966, at the age of 75. Regarding weight, Dr. Kempner wrote:

> Patients who were obese were urged to reduce. However, changes in blood sugar levels, insulin requirements, cholesterol levels, blood pressure, and so on occurred both in patients who lost weight and in those who did not have a significant weight change.... The reduction in blood pressure and heart size and the improvement ... in diabetic patients treated by the rice diet are the same as those found in non-diabetic patients with cardiovascular disease. (*W Kempner et al 1958 p 370*)

Several of the diabetic patients came with foot ulcers, another not uncommon complication, which often led to amputation. However, on the rice diet, with the improved circulation and better diabetic control, only one of our patients ever needed amputation.*

---

* I am reminded of one man, not a diabetic but with hypertensive vascular disease, who had healed so well that he resumed hunting. Unfortunately, he shot himself in the leg and had a below-knee amputation. He developed phantom-limb pain, for which additional limb reduction was advised. Our neurosurgeon, Dr. Barnes Woodhall, was passing in the corridor and Dr. Kempner asked him to have a look at the patient. Dr. Woodhall advised the patient to pat his stump, first with his hand then increasingly firmly with a reflex hammer. He explained that the stump felt pain because it missed the sensations coming up the leg from the foot's contact with the floor. The patting worked, and the man's pain was relieved without further surgery. I wonder if this simple treatment is ever used now.

# Obesity

As early as 1945, Dr. Kempner had noticed the fringe benefit of substantial weight loss in many of his patients. Although most of these early patients were not obese, many of them did arrive with excess weight. Dr. Kempner regarded obesity as a derangement of cellular metabolism. For this reason, and also because of the frequent vascular complications associated with obesity, he started treating the disorder. In 1962 he reported findings on one early group of 19 patients, ranging in age from 17 to 54 years old, who entered the program primarily because of obesity; each lost at least 100 pounds. Only three of these patients were free of vascular or metabolic disorder when admitted; the remaining 16 had hypertensive vascular disease and three of them were diabetic. Their entry weights ranged from 238 to 462 pounds. After treatment on the rice diet for an average of 33 weeks, their weights ranged from 135 to 262 pounds. At the end of treatment, all the patients were disease-free, except for one who still had impaired glucose tolerance. (*WKF Bulletin 1955 p 15*)

To handle the volume of inquiries about the rice diet and obesity, our office developed a form letter, which we called "the OOL," for Ordinary Obesity Letter. We usually managed to answer all incoming letters by the end of the day, but after the publicity surrounding Burl Ives's visit, two of the secretaries had to put in an additional ten hours or so a week, coming in at night or over the weekend. We began referring to the letters as "night OOLs" and "day OOLs."

When we started treating young patients for obesity, I doubted initially that subjecting them to the complex and expensive battery of tests developed for our kidney and heart patients would reveal anything of interest. To my surprise, examination revealed that almost all of them had some combination of decreased kidney function, decreased lung volume, large heart, high blood pressure, or diabetes mellitus, and even eyeground changes. In a later study of 106 massively obese patients who each lost more than 100 pounds, we found that these complications disappeared in nearly all cases when their weight approached normal. (*W Kempner et al 1975*)

Weight loss is not always significant in the treatment of vascular disease, however. Many rice diet patients were of normal or even low weight. A striking example is the case of a 56-year-old business man from Chicago, who came to us in 1946 for treatment of cardiac failure. At entry he weighed 123 pounds and looked, according to Dr. Kempner, like "a victim of starvation." After four months on the diet, his heart size had decreased from 19.8 centimeters to 17.9, his liver enlargement had disappeared, and, although edema was no longer present, his weight had *increased* to 141 pounds. After two and a half years on the diet, his heart size was 16.3 and his weight 138, and he looked years younger. He returned for frequent followup examinations for five years after entering the program. During his last stay he developed a urinary tract infection and died of renal failure.

There are two basic types of overweight people: those whose weight gain is related to circumstance, and those in whom it is primarily a function of their particular physiology. The great majority of our overweight early patients with vascular and kidney disease were in the former group, as are many patients who now turn to the rice diet program primarily for weight loss. These people have been busy and successful, with more money for restaurant eating and less time and inclination for exercise. They have gained their weight slowly, ten or fifteen pounds per year. Others have gained substantially, fifty to seventy-five pounds or more, during and after some crisis: pregnancy, surgery, accidents, failing relationships. Most of the people in this group have the capacity to lose weight without difficulty and to keep it off. They must learn to balance intake and output, and to sustain the effort with occasional resumption of intensive diet if they find themselves gaining more than ten pounds. And they must accept the fact that, as one ages, one needs fewer calories. The fundamental metabolism of these people has probably not been significantly disturbed.

In the second, and smaller, group of patients, obesity stems from a complex disorder that is still not fully understood but apparently combines impaired metabolism with one or more of the numerous factors that influence the brain's perception of appetite and satiety. There is no overt glandular abnormality, however, such as low thyroid metabolism or gonadal dysfunction. Obesity in these patients often starts as early as age six to eight, with seesawing weight gain and loss (mostly gain) over the patient's lifetime. These people too can lose weight relatively easily, but they rarely achieve a normal weight, and if their efforts slacken they tend to regain five to fifteen pounds in just a few days. It was and is our hope that, if these unfortunate people can manage to get to a low normal weight and maintain it for many months, their disturbed metabolism and perceptions could "reset" to the new norms and the struggle to maintain their new status would be easier. But, with a few notable exceptions, the greatly obese are fated to continue their pattern of gaining and losing.

In May 1972 Dr. Kempner wrote to an insurance company that had sought his advice regarding a claim by an obese young woman:

> The underlying factor for severe obesity is still not measurable. The dysfunction is possibly in one of the brain centers (hypothalamus area) which are not yet accessible for testing, or is a genetic factor (family trend) which also is still obscure.... Now, I would like to ask you a question: Why can so many people eat what they want and not get

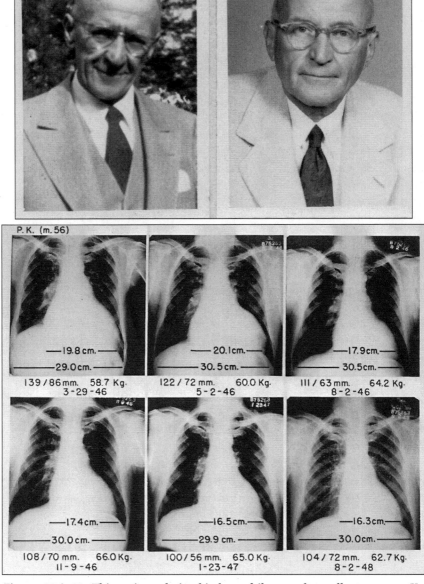

Figures 39 & 40. This patient admitted in heart failure made excellent recovery. X-rays show his heart returned to normal size, despite weight gain, and at a four-year followup, he appeared a generation younger. (At entry, left, he was 56 years old.)

fat? I think this X factor should be considered in the problem of obesity, and obesity should be accepted as a medical problem.

I think Dr. Kempner would have been most interested in the recent finding that fat itself is now considered an organ, which produces several hormones and cytokines, some of which in turn lead to further accumulation of weight.

## Arthritis

Our patients, especially the older and heavier ones, frequently arrived with osteoarthritis (degenerative joint disease), a common form of arthritis exacerbated, if not caused, by overweight, lack of exercise, and poor circulation. On the rice diet, their joint symptoms usually improved. Certainly this is in part secondary to weight loss and improved circulation; it probably is also helped by the mild exercise of walking. Some patients, instructed to lose weight preparatory to surgical treatment of their arthritis, found that after losing the weight they no longer needed the surgery. Sodium restriction also played a role by reducing the swelling in and around the joints, an important factor in reducing pain, and the weight loss decreased the mechanical strain on the joints. Increasing blood flow—and thus oxygen—to the joints supports the healing process, and has customarily been achieved by applying heat to the affected area.

Although the reasons are not clear, rheumatoid arthritis frequently remits in patients on the rice diet. One of Dr. Kempner's greatest successes with rheumatoid arthritis was with a 51-year-old woman of normal weight, who came to him with a 30-year history of arthritis. She had marked deformities and limited motion in many joints, and she was in constant pain. When her condition flared up, she could walk only with crutches. Her many attempts over the years to alleviate this condition covered a wide range: tonsillectomy, appendectomy, and tooth extraction (not uncommon at the time, when infection was considered a possible contributor to arthritis); typhoid injections and other fever therapies; thermal baths, osteopathic treatment, and autogenous blood. All were unsuccessful. Soon after beginning the rice diet, her joint pain decreased markedly and she was able to walk normally. She remained on the diet for over 20 years, during which time, except for one brief recurrence of joint pain, she was virtually symptom-free.

## Headache and Pseudotumor

There was persuasive anecdotal evidence of the beneficial effects of the rice diet on headache, including migraine. One notable example was the writer Upton Sinclair, who experienced debilitating headaches whenever he became intensely absorbed in his writing—and, as the author of some ninety books and plays, plus innumerable magazine articles, he wrote nearly daily for over six decades. He consulted doctors, nutritionists, "faddists," and therapists of all kinds without achieving relief. In an article in the December 1963 issue of *Harper's Magazine* he related how he finally found the cure. After his wife of forty years suffered a massive heart attack, she went on the rice diet, which he prepared for her every day for three or four years, during which time she steadily improved. Unfortunately, she tired of the monotony, gave up the diet, and her health steadily declined until her death. But Mr. Sinclair, impressed with the diet's effect on his wife's health, thought it might do something for his headaches as well. "Remember," he wrote in *Harper's*,

> for half a century I had been saying, 'I am never more than twenty-four hours ahead of a headache.' Now I can say: 'I have done my normal amount of writing, and I have forgotten what a headache feels like.' … I no longer play tennis, but I take care of a half-acre of flowers and foliage, and I drive downtown twice a day for mail and errands. My age is eighty-five. I have come through the ordeals of death and a new life without a trace of physical strain. To me it is a miracle: only the diet can account for it.

Some obese people occasionally suffer a debilitating condition known as *pseudotumor cerebri,* characterized by a marked increase in intracranial pressure due to accumulated fluid within the skull, but with no underlying tumor. Pseudotumor occurs mostly in young women, in whom it is almost always accompanied by menstrual abnormalities. Its cause is unknown. The pressure produces headaches, dizziness, and visual disturbance, and is usually treated by repeated lumbar punctures to remove cerebrospinal fluid or, in severe cases, surgical insertion of a drain to reroute fluid into the abdomen, where it is absorbed. Among all our patients who suffered from this condition, marked papilledema was present. Before-and-after eye photographs were available on nine patients, allowing us to document the effects of the rice diet. All of them recovered completely. One memorable case involved a 44-year-old woman, a physician, who came to the clinic weighing 348 pounds, suffering from shortness of breath, somnolence, and visual disturbance so severe that she had been forced to give up her medical practice and was no longer able to drive. After seven months on the rice diet, her eyegrounds were normal, her weight was 235, and she was able to resume her practice—and to drive herself to work.

## Psoriasis

Psoriasis, a chronic scaling, disfiguring skin condition, also responded very well to the rice diet treatment. The skin usually remained clear as long as the strict diet was maintained, but lesions often reappeared if the diet was discontinued. We did not establish whether the improvement in the psoriasis was due to an increase of a beneficial substance in the rice diet or to the decrease of a harmful one present in ordinary diets, but we suspected it was the latter. (*Newborg 1986*)

I remember Dr. Kempner telling us that one of his colleagues, a cardiology professor, had stopped him in the hall one day to profess his new confidence in the rice diet. When Dr. Kempner asked what had prompted this new enthusiasm, the doctor told him that every time his psoriasis flared up he put himself on the rice diet and found that the psoriasis disappeared in a very short while. "I don't know why it works," the doctor said, "but it works."

# Kudos and Controversy

Dr. Kempner's rice diet treatment of heart and kidney disease was a radical departure from medical orthodoxy, and his success not only in slowing or halting disease but actually in reversing its effects—results unexpected even by him—was a challenge to the establishment. However, a dietary approach to these disorders was not entirely without precedent. As early as 1922, Allen and Sherill (*Allen & Sherill 1922*) had reported obtaining positive therapeutic results in treating arterial hypertension through a sodium-restricted diet. It is unlikely that Dr. Kempner was familiar with their work, but he may well have known of Dr. Franz Volhard, a distinguished German internist who published results of similar trials in 1931.* (*Volhard 1931*) Although the earlier experimenters were on the right track, they prescribed far less sodium restriction and did not monitor patients' adherence to the regimen. Their findings, except for blood pressure measurements, were largely concerned with subjective improvement. In any case, their treatment did not attract widespread attention and seems to have made little impact. Dr. Kempner's results, by contrast, elicited a strong and mixed response from the medical establishment.

The positive effects of diet were not apparent to everyone. A book appearing several years before Dr. Kempner's Chicago presentation suggested that diet food was so unpalatable that patients simply didn't eat enough, thus reducing their metabolic rate. (*Fishberg 1939*) Commenting on Dr. Kempner's results, one skeptical paper (*Page & Corcoran 1945*) proposed that they were due not to salt

---

* On January 9, 1950, Dr. Volhard wrote to Dr. Kempner: "I am deeply impressed with your paper and I would be very thankful for a reprint. For about thirty years I have prescribed strictly salt-free food with very good success, but the success of your rice diet seems even greater. But what astonishes me is that your patients eat this monotonous diet for weeks and months and do not revolt.... Your method impresses me greatly, but even more the obedience of your patients." Dr. Kempner replied [February 2, 1950], "Motivating the patients to follow the rice diet strictly is not always easy. During their first three or four months here in Durham, most of them are under daily supervision. This continues to some degree after their departure, through periodic urine analyses for sodium chloride, etc. Patients who have had the most serious manifestations in the heart and eyegrounds follow the diet best. With diabetics, it came out that not only do they tolerate the diet well but the amount of insulin had to be reduced." (*W Kempner 1954b p 329*)

restriction but simply to "rest in bed and the psychotherapy of constant attention." Another attempt to explain away the benefits of the rice diet was to at-
tribute them to simple starvation. Dr. Kempner pointed out the "fundamental
chemical differences between the effects of starvation and of the rice diet":

> ... hemoglobin, red blood cells, calcium, and total protein, A/G ratio,
> sugar, carbohydrate tolerance, and $CO_2$-combining power in the blood
> are decreased in starvation. On the rice diet, they are unchanged or
> increased. The blood non-protein nitrogen and urea nitrogen are in-
> creased in starvation. On the rice diet, they are decreased. Blood vol-
> ume and interstitial fluid volume are unchanged or increased in
> starvation. On the rice diet, they are decreased. The nitrogen balance
> is negative in starvation. On the rice diet, it is in equilibrium. (*W
> Kempner 1951b p 2*)

Those who came to see for themselves were more convinced. The doctor of
a Canadian patient who had made an impressive recovery came to see Dr.
Kempner's clinic, I recall, and reported on his visit to his medical society. When
his colleagues asked, "Weren't these results due to Dr. Kempner's personality?"
he replied, "I saw the rats in their cages, and I don't think they were a bit impressed with his personality." A good many doctors made serious attempts to
apply his methods. A few of them were successful, and their study reports and
correspondence with Dr. Kempner convey some of the intense interest stirred
up by publication of his work.

On April 10, 1945, two months after the North Carolina Medical Journal had
published Dr. Kempner's lengthy report, which JAMA and the Archives of Internal Medicine had rejected because of the attendant controversy, the Journal's
assistant editor wrote to Dr. Kempner:

> I wish you could hear the controversial comments on the subject of the
> rice diet that I get with my lunch every day (the comments, not the
> diet) and witness the gradual conversion of some of our most cynical
> scoffers. One of them, who told me three months ago that it was all
> bosh and poppycock, thinks now that he may write an article on it
> himself after he gets a small series of patients to report on. Another
> is writing you for a reprint.... All of which should help a little to res-
> cue you from that early grave you predicted.

Dr. Aaron H. Kallet, of Syracuse, New York, who was physician to Harvey
M. Smith, of the Smith-Corona typewriter company, one of Dr. Kempner's
early notable successes, wrote Dr. Kempner on June 29, 1945:

I am happy to report that Mr. Harvey M. Smith's blood pressure is 148/90. That is slightly higher than the last examination but he has changed his residence and is in the process of moving which I believe is a factor. He is feeling fine and I know you will be pleased with his condition when you see'him within the next few weeks....

I am treating a large number of patients along the lines you are following and am thrilled with the results. Two and a half weeks ago I saw a man forty-eight years old, weighing 287 pounds, systolic pressure 244, diastolic 130, with a persistent tachycardia. He came to me shortly after being checked by his company's physician, a cardiologist, with a report of a very serious basic condition. Within two weeks he lost 17 pounds, blood pressure dropped to 148 systolic, with 96 diastolic and a pulse rate down to 86. Except for feeling weak he said he hadn't felt as well in years. I am obtaining gratifying results with practically every case that will cooperate.

Guided only by Dr. Kempner's initial published findings, a Miami physician, Dr. Jay Flipse, put some of his own patients on the rice diet, and by November 1946 he was able to report that his strict rice and fruit routine had successfully controlled blood pressure in 20 of 32 patients, although, as he pointed out, "the diet is difficult for patients to follow and many failures result from poor cooperation." (*Flipse & Flipse 1947*) But Dr. Flipse kept at it, and evidently was more successful than most in maintaining rigor in the diet and discipline among his patients. In March 1960 he reported:

> The diet of Dr. Kempner, in which the fat and sodium were markedly restricted, not only controlled hypertension but also caused a reversal of the atherosclerotic changes in the retinal vessels. This astounding demonstration of the reversibility of the process of atherosclerosis has warranted the hope that some program may be devised which will not only prevent an extension of the disease but also cause a reversal of at least part of the damage that has already been done. (*Flipse 1960*)

Many of Dr. Kempner's would-be imitators, however, demonstrated an amazing degree of ignorance of the principles on which the rice diet was based. In a letter of January 1945 Dr. Kempner reported to Dr. Hanes, "At the moment we have a patient who was put on the rice diet by Longcope (at Johns Hopkins Hospital). He ate it very faithfully but was allowed some additional ham, pork, and fish." Another doctor wrote to Dr. Kempner that he was giving his patient egg three times a week, to break up the diet's monotony. When a group of doctors in Boston tried the diet on six of their patients, one patient complained that she had been disturbed all night by dreams of drowning in rice; the doctors found this sufficient reason to suspend the diet.

Along with the widespread underestimation of the importance of strict observance, there was the fact that few doctors had the necessary laboratory facilities for the degree of monitoring required. Doctors whose clinics lacked the equipment for such "microanalysis" found it difficult, if not impossible, to gauge accurately the patients' adherence to the diet. And without accurate and frequent analysis of serum electrolytes, some patients could get into serious trouble. At Washington University in St. Louis, one of six patients being treated with the rice diet died because his sodium deficiency was not detected and treated early enough. The doctor had failed to monitor his electrolytes. Dr. Kempner had not fully anticipated, in developing the rice diet, how difficult it would be to maintain the necessary rigor in its administration. In January 1942, declining an invitation to discuss his diet at a medical meeting, he had written, "I should not like to speak about it before I can summarize my ideas ... in a few simple rules which can easily be followed by the practitioner." [WK to O. Norris Smith, 1/27/42] But mounting evidence convinced Dr. Kempner that the rice diet could not be administered except by staff trained by him and familiar with the chemical intricacies of the diet and its potential hazards. Dr. Kempner also pointed out another vulnerability of the rice diet:

> The apparent simplicity of the rice diet has not infrequently proved a handicap. We have seen patients who had been treated with the diet just because the manometer had shown blood pressure figures above normal, and in whom tumors, infections, etc. had been overlooked. (W Kempner 1948a p 560)

Unaffected by the clamor (except for the huge increase in his patient load), Dr. Kempner continued to work with his patients and in the laboratory, and to make his results known. His second major presentation was on January 15, 1946, this time to the New York Academy of Medicine. There, he responded to several of his critics' charges:

> The consensus of opinion at the present time is that dietary treatment is useful in kidney disease, but of little or no value in hypertension without obvious renal involvement. Goldring and Chasis, in 1944, summed up the prevalent view in their book on hypertension: "The diet in uncomplicated hypertension requires no essential change from the normal." ... Those who question the value of diet in the treatment of hypertensive vascular disease say that in those patients who responded to our diet our diagnosis was probably incorrect. I think that

in most cases the differential diagnosis presents no difficulties. (*W Kempner 1946 pp 360, 365*)

Addressing the charge of incorrect diagnosis, Dr. Kempner pointed out that most of his patients came to him with long-standing and already well-documented histories of disease. He cited the case of a 42-year-old patient whom he treated for benign essential hypertension. Between March 1940 and November 1941, the man had been seen in three different New York hospitals with blood pressure as high as 200 systolic and 125 to 140 diastolic. On his doctor's recommendation, he had a Smithwick sympathectomy, at that time the most popular treatment for severe hypertension, which in his case was not helpful. In March 1945 the patient came to Dr. Kempner, who put him on a 1500-calorie diet. When the restricted diet had made no appreciable change in his blood pressure after twenty days, Dr. Kempner started him on the rice diet, and after one month his blood pressure was 129/94. I am not certain why the patient was not started immediately on the rice diet, but probably, in the absence of significant complications from hypertension, Dr. Kempner felt he might respond to less rigorous treatment.

Four years later, with continued diet and no medication, the patient's blood pressure was 114/82. For an additional two years he continued to follow the diet more or less strictly, but then he began to relax his control and after six years abandoned all dietary restriction. His weight rose from 183 to 220 pounds; however, his disease apparently had healed and did not recur. Nine years after admission, he remarked to Dr. Kempner, "Doctor, I have really eaten like a pig, but I promise that I will not do it again." Dr. Kempner answered, "Your blood pressure is normal, your heart size and electrocardiogram are normal. Perhaps it is all right now for you to eat like a pig." However, they did agree that the weight should be reduced and that fat and salt should be restricted. (*W Kempner 1954a p 87*) The patient lived an additional eight years after this conversation.

Not all patients were successful in maintaining the discipline necessary for success; some gave up altogether, others relaxed the restrictions bit by bit. For the most part, their condition did not respond well to a less strict regimen. A sad example was a 60-year-old patient who first came in 1946 with arteriosclerosis of the kidneys, which had led to heart failure.

> He had been treated with a salt-restricted diet, digitalis, potassium nitrate, theobromine, and mercurials. In spite of this, his heart had become progressively larger, and the signs and symptoms of cardiac failure had increased. When all the drugs except digitalis were discontinued and the salt-poor diet replaced by the strict rice diet, his heart became decidedly smaller and all the signs and symptoms of

cardiac failure disappeared. As long as he had any discomfort, he adhered strictly to the rice diet, but the better he felt the more careless he grew, making additions of his own choice. After some time, all his former symptoms would gradually return, and each time this happened he would come back here to make a fresh start on the strict regimen. When the salt figure decreased, his heart became smaller in size; when the salt figure increased, the heart became larger again. This pattern repeated itself for six years, until finally the heart failure was no longer reversible. The weight of the heart at autopsy was 900 grams [it should be less than 350]. (*W Kempner 1954a p 87*)

In another case, a 40-year-old patient with a clear prior diagnosis of benign essential hypertension came to Dr. Kempner in February 1948. Despite a long history of treatment, including a Smithwick sympathectomy, her blood pressure on admission was 222/131. She was put on the rice diet, but after six months it had had very little effect: her blood pressure was 212/121; moreover, a cottony exudate had developed in her eye, indicating that vascular disease was progressing. Even a year later, while the exudate had disappeared, her blood pressure was still 192/126. Although she thought she was following the rice diet strictly when she was away from Durham, her urine at such times showed unacceptable concentrations of chlorides. Dr. Kempner was convinced that she would eventually respond to treatment, if she could just persevere— and if he could keep her under close observation to ward off dangerous side effects of such prolonged dieting. She moved to Durham permanently, took a job, and kept faithfully to the diet. After two years on the diet her blood pressure had declined only slightly, to 180/104, but she felt well enough to take on a more active job with a good deal of responsibility, involving constant travel. It took nearly two more years to get her blood pressure down to normal; in the first three months of 1953, it averaged 120/76. Meanwhile, after the first three years, her diet was modified in small increments to increase variety, with no adverse effects. After five years, her blood pressure was normal. On the modified rice diet, she lived well until 1995, when she died of complications from smoking, which she was unable and unwilling to give up.

Dr. Kempner was criticized for not conducting baseline studies prior to treatment. This was not entirely justified, as some of his published studies included baseline measurements for a week or more prior to beginning the rice diet. Dr. Kempner replied to his critics that, as heart disease at that time was the number one killer in America and patients with malignant hypertension had a life expectancy of only three to six months, to delay treatment of these patients for even a short period in order to get base-line figures seemed unnecessary at best, if not indeed criminal. An article in the Walter Kempner Foundation Bulletin addressed this issue, with the example of a 20-year-old patient with malignant hypertension, advanced eyeground disease, and a history of convulsions. She had been admitted to Duke Hospital and started immediately on the rice diet by the intern.

> When Dr. Kempner and his associates made hospital rounds the next morning, Dr. Kempner asked the 14 physicians and students present whether the intern had acted correctly by starting treatment without getting all studies completed first, and without an initial test period of at least one to two weeks to establish a more objective baseline. Dr. Kempner's Research Fellow at that time, a very well-trained and competent physician who had been a lieutenant colonel in the Canadian medical corps in World War II, said emphatically that it had been very unscientific on the part of the intern to institute treatment so prematurely. The intern argued back that the patient's condition was critical, that the convulsions and blindness afforded enough evidence of the extent of the disease, and that she might easily die during such a "control time" if it were to be enforced. Dr. Kempner kept a poker face and said: "Since we are living here in a democratic country, we'd better get a vote on the subject." The vote was eleven in favor of the intern, three in favor of the research fellow. Without changing his expression, Dr. Kempner turned to the three and said, "I suppose we have to follow the decision of the majority in this case. And as a matter of fact, if I were the patient myself, Dr. X (the intern) would be my choice too." (*WKF Bulletin 1972 p 15*)

This straightforward approach to teaching as well as to his research and clinical practice won Dr. Kempner the admiration of many interns, as well. One of them, John Verner, once wrote to me:

> I remember vividly a lesson taught by Dr. K. He had a patient on the private service and he requested that I digitalize [administer digitalis to combat heart failure] the patient. Being a hardheaded intern, I replied that I did not digitalize patients who were not in heart failure or having any arrhythmia. He smiled and dropped the subject. That night, I was awakened about 4 a.m. after about two hours of sleep, called to the bedside of the same patient, now in pulmonary edema. Recovery was achieved with rapid IV digitalization and diuretics. The next morning [Dr. Kempner] smiled again and said simply, "You learn now, young doctor." There was no rebuke, just good-natured humor. [October 2004]

From his expanding patient base, Dr. Kempner continued to offer the medical and scientific establishment increasing evidence of the rice diet's effect. In 1947, he twice addressed the American College of Physicians, at their March meeting at the Mayo Clinic and then at their November meeting at Massachusetts General Hospital. In October, he addressed the Scientific Assembly of the Medical Society of the District of Columbia. Over the next couple of years there were presentations in Atlanta, Williamsburg, Pittsburgh, and New York. In 1950, he addressed the First International Conference on Cardiology in Paris, and in 1951, the Pan-American Ophthalmological Society in Miami. He never explained why, after this last appearance, he stopped making presentations at professional meetings, but I think he felt the information was now widely available and he wanted to concentrate his time and energy on patients.

As the evidence of his success accumulated and was disseminated, Dr. Kempner continued to win converts. For example, in 1939, in his major textbook on hypertension and nephritis, Dr. A. M. Fishberg had stated his conviction that rigid salt restriction in patients with essential hypertension was not of sufficient benefit to warrant its general use. (*Fishberg 1939*) By 1958, however, he had changed his tune:

> I believe firmly, much more firmly than I did a few years ago, in the value of sodium restriction.... I have come to think it is of tremendous importance. Sodium must be restricted to less than 500 mg per day before there is any chance of demonstrable lowering of the blood pressure within a relatively short period of time. I now also believe that lesser degrees of sodium restriction may slow the progress of hypertensive disease.... So-called malignant hypertension is disappearing.... The only way I can account for [this] is because of something that we have done in recent years. Today, practically every patient with elevated blood pressure is receiving a sodium-restricted diet. (*Fishberg 1958 p 722*)

One notable physician intrigued by Dr. Kempner's reports was Dr. Paul Dudley White of Harvard, a pioneering cardiologist noted for his advocacy of fitness and exercise for healthy hearts. He became a celebrity in the 1950s as the physician who successfully treated President Eisenhower's infarct. In an article on his investigations into diet and the management of hypertension, White wrote:

> Because of the considerable experience during the past four or five years of Dr. Kempner of Duke University at Durham, North Carolina,

in the treatment of hypertensive patients with a strict rice diet and because of his reported success in a good many cases I myself made a pilgrimage to his clinic a month ago, saw some of his cases, and had a sample rice meal at one of the rice houses in town. Kemper introduced this diet some seven or eight years ago in the treatment of patients with renal disease and insufficiency because of both low protein and low sodium content and of the easily assimilated protein in the rice itself.... [I]n many patients such limitation after they become accustomed to it and if they are willing to stick it out does not seem to cause any particular hardship, and light or even average work can be resumed without trouble. It is reported that about two-thirds of those hypertensive patients who are willing to give this diet a fair trial are distinctly helped by it subjectively and in blood pressure levels, and in some cases cardiac enlargement and eyeground abnormalities decrease or clear away and the electrocardiogram improves. Thus hypertensive heart disease has been proved to be reversible by the rice diet. (*White 1947 p 740*)

Following his visit Dr. White twice invited Dr. Kempner to Boston to lecture on his work.

The medical profession's reception was favorable in general, but not unanimously so. Other physicians' chief difficulty was with replicating his results, because it was so difficult to persuade patients to keep to the strict diet. In February 1949, an editorial in the New England Journal of Medicine addressed this aspect of the treatment:

Dietary restriction of one sort or another has been utilized in the treatment of hypertensive disease for many years. In 1945 Kempner presented the details of his commendably aggressive approach to the dietary treatment of this group of diseases and thereby stirred up a great deal of comment, both medical and lay. Kempner's own therapeutic results are little short of miraculous and have justifiably impressed numerous competent and critical observers who have visited the North Carolina clinic. Investigators other than Kempner have obtained favorable, but not miraculous, results in most cases, and the chief difficulty seems to center around the extreme monotony of the diet. Most physicians lack the extraordinary persuasive powers required to keep a patient eating rice and certain types of fruit for weeks, months or even indefinitely. The usual result is that the patient fails to eat all the food presented to him and, not infrequently, finally rejects the diet altogether....

Kempner finds that patients receiving the diet lose weight initially but after some weeks the weight becomes stable and all is well—in fact, so well that the diet can often be modified slightly. He attributes the initial loss of weight to loss of fluid. It has proved very difficult for other investigators to confirm or deny these claims, mainly because so many patients cannot conform to the rigid requirements of the Kempner regimen over long periods. It seems clear, however, that patients receiving the Kempner regimen in clinics other than Kempner's own lose not only fluid but also body tissue.... Salt restriction in such patients is unquestionably highly important. Reduction in weight over and above that due to fluid accumulation is crucial in many obese patients with cardiac failure. Heretofore the patient has been offered a low-calorie diet, which often supplies 800 calories or less, to achieve loss of body tissue. He has been implored and cajoled not to eat more than the allowed amount, in spite of which he often reaches a point where he secretly takes extra food and the physician cannot understand why the patient's weight remains too high. The psychologic, as well as the physiologic, advantages of the Kempner regimen in this situation seem not to have been appreciated. Using the rice-fruit diet, the physician, instead of pleading with his patient to eat less, actually has to urge the patient to eat all the food given him. The very low salt intake, a difficult feature to control on any sort of hospital diet other than that devised by Kempner, helps to rid the patient of excessive fluid, and concurrently, the usual inability to maintain the caloric intake allowed by the Kempner regimen causes a reduction in body fat and protein. Practically speaking, there probably is no more effective diet for obese decompensated cardiac patients.

Although the Kempner regimen is certainly not the final answer in the treatment of hypertensive disease, it is an important development in the search for a practical and uniformly successful method of treating the disorder. Furthermore, it may well find a permanent place in the treatment of some types of congestive cardiac failure and even in uncomplicated obesity.

Doubt persisted about the authenticity of the eyeground photographs, which offered the most surprising and the most significant evidence that hypertensive and diabetic retinopathy could be reversed. Regarding these, Kempner later recalled:

It was the eyeground photographs more than anything else that bothered those who had insisted that diet was of no value in the treatment of hypertensive vascular disease. Since eyegrounds are as individual as fingerprints and the photographs compared, therefore, were obviously of the same patient, some people actually went so far as to accuse us of having reversed the dates, intimating that the pictures of the normal eyegrounds were the first ones and those of the abnormal eyegrounds had been taken later. (*W Kempner 1954a p 91*)

Dr. Banks Anderson, chief of ophthalmology at Duke, who defended Kempner's findings against skeptics, had been thoroughly convinced by his own observation of many of Dr. Kempner's patients. Two patients in particular had extensive papilledema which he thought must surely be due to expanding intracranial lesions; in both instances, however, their response to the rice diet showed that the entire picture was caused by malignant hypertension. When Dr. Anderson saw these patients again after some months on the rice diet, he wrote in his consultation notes,

> [regarding the first patient] This patient's eye grounds are improved to an unbelievable degree. I have never previously seen such an extensive papilledema subside with such minimal retinal scarring, nor for that matter do I think I have ever seen a patient with this degree of hypertensive retinopathy alive after this period of time…. [regarding the second patient] Review of notes indicates that when I saw this patient last I was of the opinion that the papilledema was too great to have been due exclusively to hypertension. I was wrong. Fundoscopic examination through the undilated pupils shows no evidence of papilledema at this time … [T]here are no areas of exudate, hemorrhage, or pigmentation. (*W Kempner 1954a p 90*)

Taking note of ongoing efforts by other physicians and researchers to isolate the active principle of the rice diet, variously thought to be sodium restriction (*Grollman & Harrison 1945*), protein restriction (*Selye & Stone 1946*), or cholesterol reduction (*Dock 1946*),* Dr. Kempner continually stressed the necessity for these multiple and severe restrictions, which he sometimes referred to as "total war." In presenting case histories in his publications he drove the point home that, regardless of the governing principle at work, it could not be successful without continued scrupulous adherence.

---

* I also remember hearing of some speculation at that time about the beneficial role of the rice diet's high potassium content, which has been stressed in a recent publication. (*Hawkins 2006*)

In his 1949 paper, Dr. Kempner summed up ten years of experience with the rice diet:

> The treatment of heart and kidney disease and of hypertensive and arteriosclerotic vascular disease with the rice diet is either ineffective or dangerous unless it is done under rigidly controlled conditions. Ineffective, because small or "minimal" additions to the diet may spoil the entire therapeutic result; dangerous, because a strict observance of the diet may lead to a deficiency of vitally important elements unless care is taken that the equilibrium between intake and loss of these substances is maintained. For both reasons, therefore, continuous supervision over a long period of time, including constant checks of blood and urine chemistry, is essential.
>
> Rigidly controlled conditions are likewise indispensable for evaluation of the therapeutic results. Claims of positive or negative results based on nothing but the blood pressure readings for four to eight weeks, before and after treatment, and not substantiated by heart films, electrocardiograms, eyeground photographs, and chemical findings, do not contribute much to the solution of this problem....
>
> Ten years ago, I used to teach, what was generally taught and is still written in textbooks published as late as 1947, that the presence of advanced neuroretinopathy in malignant hypertension is an ominous prognostic sign indicative of the terminal stage of an irreparable disease. My experience with the rice diet has taught me that not only can so-called benign hypertensive vascular disease be effectively treated even when critical complications are present, but also that malignant hypertension, in spite of advanced neuroretinopathy, may either be changed into the benign form of hypertension or made to disappear completely. *The important result is not that the change in the course of the disease has been achieved by the rice diet, but that the course of the disease can be changed.* [emphasis the author's] (*W Kempner 1949b p 821, 856*)

When he presented this paper to the annual conference of the American College of Physicians at the Waldorf-Astoria in New York, on March 30, 1949, he received a standing ovation. The chairman of the session commented, "When Dr. Kempner came to this country, it was a great loss for Germany and a tremendous gain for the United States!"

# The Rice Houses

As Dr. Kempner's reputation grew, many prospective patients—some of them in the late stages of disease—were unable to get appointments; patients routinely had to wait several months, or even a year, for the first available opening. Regrettably, we occasionally received letters like the following (May 1948):

Dear Sir, On your list of appointments you have the name of my Mother to take your treatment for high blood pressure.... Her appointment with you was for August 19th, 1948. [She] was taken by death very suddenly on May 9 of this year. Her high blood pressure caused a stroke and a cerebral hemorrhage. I thought perhaps if I gave you this information, another person could have the appointment you had given her, and perhaps save someone's life. I will appreciate it if you could cancel the room reservation at the hotel for me. Yours truly,

A great many requests, from both doctors and lay persons, asked for detailed instructions on following the diet at home. There was no easy answer to these requests, to which Dr. Kempner replied promptly, courteously, and firmly. To potential patients he wrote,

I am sorry that I cannot be of immediate help to you, but I am sure you will understand that I cannot give any advice without having had an opportunity to examine you and to study your case.

If, at any time, you could arrange to come here without too much inconvenience, I should be glad to see you. Please let me know some months in advance so that I may make an appointment for you.

To physicians who inquired, he was happy to send reprints of his articles, always with the caveat that, as he wrote in another paper, the diet

is either ineffective or dangerous unless it is done under rigidly controlled conditions. Ineffective because small or minimal additions to the diet may spoil the entire therapeutic result; dangerous, because a strict observance of the diet may lead to a deficiency of vitally important elements unless care is taken that the equilibrium between intake and loss of these substances is maintained. (*W Kempner 1949b p 821*)

For the eligible patients who did manage to be accepted for treatment, there were several technical problems in handling the volume of work. To keep track of all the data generated by the many and frequent laboratory tests, Dr. Kempner devised a streamlined method of handling patient data to replace traditional bulky medical histories. Moreover, the rising number of patients also created a problem of where to lodge and feed them. At that time Duke Hospital had seventy beds for medical patients, divided among thirteen physicians. Seven beds were allotted to Dr. Kempner, a relatively generous share but wholly inadequate to his patient load. The beginning of a solution came in late 1943 from Mrs. Walter Newton of Durham, the widow of a former patient who had died in a car accident. Mrs. Newton suggested to Dr. Kempner that she provide room and board to his patients in her house. After years of caring for her husband, she was entirely familiar with the preparation and administration of the rice diet, she now had time and rooms to spare, and she needed the money. Soon four rice patients were housed and fed in her house on Shawnee Street, where Dr. Kempner and his medical staff examined them daily and maintained strict supervision of operations. I often accompanied him on these rounds. This arrangement worked very well for everyone but did not entirely solve the housing problem. In 1945, Mrs. George Smith, a practical nurse who had worked at Duke, started a second rice house in her residence on Buchanan Street.

Accommodations at the Smith house were primitive, with three or four patients in one bedroom sharing an adjoining bathroom with one or two patients in another. These rice houses must have been a substantial culture shock to the patients coming to Durham from many parts of the world, most of whom were wealthy and accustomed to a great deal of comfort and privacy. But, confronting the imminent threat of heart attacks, strokes, and even death, these people had a driving desire to get well, and they knew that, spartan though it was, the treatment worked.

In 1946, Mrs. Newton expanded her enterprise by purchasing another property, at 1111 North Mangum Street, to be run as a rice house. Normally she housed from four to ten patients there, with many more coming for three daily meals. In 1948, Mrs. Smith moved from Buchanan to a larger and more accommodating house—first to 1017 Gloria Avenue, later to 1011 Lamond Street. She ran her rice house until 1952. The local paper described her operation in a feature article ("Mrs. Smith's Rice House—'A Dream Come True,'" Durham Morning Herald, 3/5/1950]:

The rambling, comfortable house is devoted entirely to the patients. "Smitty," her husband and grandson, George Meeks, live in the small house behind the main one. Patients eat in the dining and breakfast room at separate tables, each seating four, and the library has been turned into an examining room for the convenience of the patients who are checked every morning by Duke Hospital physicians.

"Smitty" is assisted in her work by Mrs. Hazel Vickers; Miss Benie Stebbins; Mrs. Emma Sanders, a Negro nurse who has been with her since the beginning; four maids and two waiters. Her usual pace is a steady trot, but she is never too busy to look out for the comfort and pleasure of the patients. She is always delighted to welcome them back "home" when they return for rechecks several months after dismissal. "Smitty" has a cosmopolitan group under her wing, indeed, for the patients come from such places as Africa, Latin America, the Isle of Cypress [sic] and, of course, from all over this country.

Having been referred to Dr. Kempner by Duke Hospital in 1945 because she was eager to start an eating and convalescent home for his patients, she started getting some almost before she was ready for them. Recalling the first few hectic months, she related how she had borrowed beds from an undertaker, had done all her own cooking, and felt with those first three patients that she was the busiest woman in town. Now she houses eight, feeds anywhere from 38 to 80.

.... During the war, she recalled, it was a real problem to round up all the rice and canned fruits that she needed in large amounts for her "ricers." The grocers were very helpful, she smiled gratefully. "Smitty" grinds her own rice flour out of which she prepares her own especially devised saltless, fatless, eggless recipes for cakes, and candies that usually adorn the tables on holidays, along with suitable cheery decorations.

"Smitty" has indeed made a home away from home for a handful of people, as well as being in a business which she truly enjoys and feels is useful.

"You might say I have so many children I don't know what to do, but I love them all," she beamed, "and I'm having a wonderful time. They are my family and are always welcome—as long as they stay out of the kitchen!"

The records for Mrs. Smith's and Mrs. Newton's two rice house operations show the growth of the daily patient load (for meals, not lodging). From 40 patients in 1945 and 76 in 1946, the number climbed steadily, to 164 in 1948 and, at our highest census, 330 patients in June 1970.

The article quoted above mentions the difficulties of acquiring rice diet food under wartime rationing. In fact, during and well after World War II (until at least 1947), Dr. Kempner had to submit medical requests on behalf of many of his patients for special extensions of their food rations, especially sugar. In addition, he requested major sugar exemptions for the rice houses.* The rice diet's reputation was persuasion enough. The chief of sugar rationing for North Carolina wrote Dr. Kempner (April 16, 1946):

> As you know, the writer has been very interested in the treatment of hypertensive retinopathy and has made every effort to cooperate with you in securing the proper amounts of sugar for your patients.
>
> We wonder if you have been securing good cooperation from the other areas. At several meetings in Atlanta I have made appeals for prompt handling of your applications and stated that under no circumstances should the amount be cut down. I have seen the effects on some of your patients where they have been unable to secure sugar and have had to break the diet. This is very unpleasant to us; and if there are any points which you feel are not giving you proper support, we would like very much to know them and will personally take up the matter to see if we cannot either speed up your applications or get the full amount requested.

Along with the increased load of rice diet patients scattered around Durham came the need for more staff, and of a different kind. We needed people not necessarily with medical training but knowledgeable about and committed to Dr. Kempner's program. They were to talk with patients and report to the physicians any medical problems, encourage patients on the diet, and generally help with the larger and smaller concerns of unhealthy people adapting to life in a strange town. Dr. Schlayer, Mrs. Eadie, and I were among the first to fill this function of "patient counselors." We also fielded questions about diet changes, monitored blood pressures, weighed patients, and did what one assistant called "morale-building." The occasional medical emergency that arose was handled by one of Dr. Kempner's physician associates—Dr. Starke, Dr. Peschel, or me—or by the Duke Hospital emergency room. The important role of the patient counselors caught the eye of Dr. Eugene Stead, who later developed the nation's first physician assistant program at Duke, based in part on his observations of how valuable such staff could be in a busy practice.

--------

* For British patients on the rice diet, similar requests were made of the rationing board in England, where wartime shortages were even more severe. Their response was equally cooperative.

With the expanded staff, the establishment of the rice houses, and the fast-growing patient population, Dr. Kempner's program took on the character of a sanatorium, though quite different in some respects. The rice houses provided housing for only a small percentage of the patients, usually the sickest and the youngest, who normally would have been hospitalized, not because they needed bed rest but because of the need for constant supervision. Other patients found accommodation in nearby hotels and rooming houses, rented apartments or houses, or even occasionally stayed in trailer parks. With their sleeping quarters scattered throughout Durham, the patients came together daily at the rice houses for meals and medical oversight.

Seven days a week, the medical staff met with and evaluated every patient. Beginning at 6:30 in the morning, Dr. Kempner would make his rounds to see the patients. At the rice houses, two or more patient counselors would have set up "stations" around a bed, a bench, or a couch, where reclining blood pressure and other vital statistics could be measured. There were six such stations in the Mangum Street house, in two large living rooms converted for the purpose. While the patients waited their turn with the counselors, who took daily measurements and provided encouragement and advice where indicated, Dr. Kempner circulated among them chatting and checking their progress. Sometimes he would sit and address the patients more formally as a group. He gave them updates on his research and other medical news, and he taught and encouraged them, often using parables. He would point out the most successful patients as examples to the others—in his words, "forcing them down the throats" of those who complained that the diet was too strict to maintain. His talks were very popular. Dr. Kempner once made the wry observation that if people saw one road sign pointing to paradise and another pointing to a lecture on it, most of them would go to the lecture!

Before the rice houses centralized the location of rounds, Dr. Kempner went to the patients in their housing around town. I remember many dawns driving with him on these visits, a pile of patient charts on my lap. As we traveled, he would ask me for each patient's latest urine findings, to check how well they were adhering to the diet and how well their kidney disease was progressing. On these morning review sessions, Dr. Kempner said, I "acted like a lens" for him. His recall of each patient's figures was astonishing; he remembered them better than I did, even though they were measurements that, usually, I had made myself in the laboratory. We would let ourselves in and go directly to the rooms, where the patients were usually still in bed. At first, Dr. Kempner had thought it was better to examine his ambulatory patients before they got up in the morning, when their physiological state was closer to that of hospital in-patients and the findings would thus be more standardized. As the numbers grew, how-

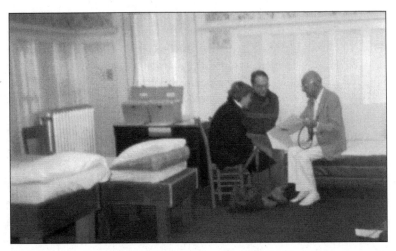

Figure 41. Dr. Kempner talking with patients at a "station" in the Mangum Street rice house. Boxes containing the all-important yellow charts at left.

ever, this routine became increasingly cumbersome and time-consuming. The daily gathering of all ambulatory patients at the rice houses was a much easier arrangement; moreover, since walking several miles daily was an integral part of the treatment program, this gave patients a good opportunity for exercise.

Because all the patients came together for mealtimes at the rice houses, a real sense of community arose among them, and enduring friendships developed among people from very different walks of life. There were even a few marriages. I remember a group of four couples who always arranged their returns to Durham at the same time, and occasionally took vacations and trips together. Two other couples who became friends chose to make their annual returns together in May, so they could attend graduation ceremonies at the surrounding universities and hear commencement addresses by famous people.

A typical day for a ricer began with a walk to the rice house for breakfast and medical checkup, then a walk to the YMCA or other facility for exercise, and a walk back for a rice house lunch. Among the more active, afternoons included group exercise such as volleyball, badminton, bowling, tennis, golf, or swimming. Others might play board games, or attend local cultural events. As other fitness programs sprang up around Durham, ricers occasionally competed with patients from those facilities. Movies and card games were staple activities. One patient from Hollywood, a director I believe, organized the ricers to perform an elaborate skit, with costumes and makeup. Similar but far less elaborate performances were occasionally organized by other patients. When a rising young opera star came to Durham for the rice diet, she performed twice for the patients.

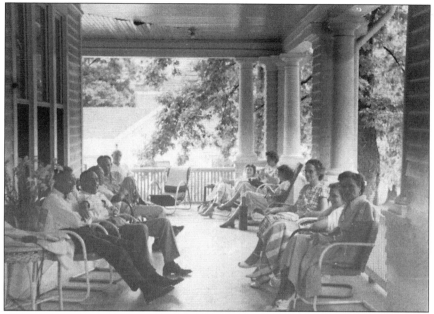

Figure 42. Patients socializing on the porch at Mangum Street.

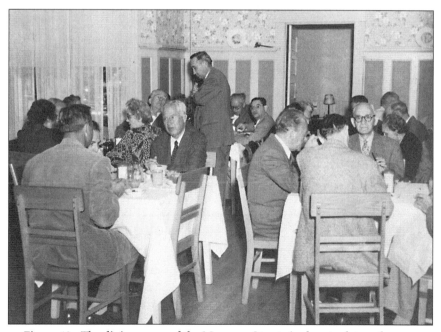

Figure 43. The dining room of the Mangum Street rice house, date unknown.

Shopping was always very popular. As patients lost weight, they required new clothes. Some patients purchased automobiles while in Durham. To celebrate his return to health on the rice diet, one of them bought a Cadillac for *each* of his four daughters. These temporary residents made a real impact on Durham's economy. The local press called Dr. Kempner "Durham's One-Man Industry," noting that his patients annually added as much as $1.8 million to the city's coffers. The city government was well aware of their debt to Dr. Kempner and his patients. One morning in 1979, the mayor and the city manager came to the Mangum Street rice house and, with a brief speech applauded by the ricers and staff gathered in the dining room, they presented Dr. Kempner with "the key to the city," actually a piece of lucite in the shape of North Carolina, with a bicentennial medallion embedded in its center.

It was not long before the success of the rice house system and its measurable effect on the local economy began to draw entrepreneurial attention. In the late nineteen-forties and fifties, letters poured in from proprietors of hotels, restaurants, spas, and clinics around the country eager to jump on the bandwagon. They usually wanted to discuss plans to convert their facilities, wholly or in part, for use as rice diet centers. Over and over Dr. Kempner replied, courteously but briefly: "The project certainly sounds very interesting. But I do not think that it will be suitable for my purposes. With many thanks for your kind offer." "I should be glad to explain to you why it is impossible for the time being to make such arrangements as you suggest...." "There are a good many problems involved which should not be overlooked...."

Rice companies offered to supply us with rice in return for endorsements of a particular brand; canned food companies offered to create modified versions of their products. The owner of the Dunkin' Donuts chain, a rice patient, even appealed to Dr. Kempner for permission to manage a national franchise of rice houses. This deliciously incongruous proposal passed quickly into rice house legend. Needless to say, Kempner was not interested in this proposal—or in most of the others.

A few well-organized and large-scale plans did gain his interest for a while. In 1948 a Mr. Kufferman, a patient from South Orange, New Jersey, apparently combining a nose for a good business deal with a genuine impulse to support the program, offered to build a comprehensive rice facility in Durham at his own expense. The proposed building would initially house the rice diet kitchens, offices, and clinic; eventually, through phased expansion, it would include patient housing as well. Dr. Kempner was of course always wary of any arrangement that would dilute his control over the administration and monitoring of the treatment. However, Kufferman seems to have managed to secure his confidence, as several drafts exist of letters of agreement drawn up over Dr. Kempner's name between February and April 1948. Of the many proposals he received over the years, this is the only such plan that seems actually to have won his approval. The latest draft available, dated April 16, reads in part as follows:

> I agree that if you acquire or begin to build such structure within four months and devote the same to the purposes stated above, you will have my full cooperation and endorsement as follows:
>
> After you or your operating company advise me you are equipped to serve to my patients the diets referred to above, I will refer to your dining room an average of two out of every three persons whom I thereafter accept as out-patients. I will encourage this ratio of new patients and many of the ones who return for reexamination to have their meals at your establishment. I must, however, require that the charge to be made for the rice and fruit diet shall not exceed $25.00 per week or $1.25 per meal, unless and until I consent in writing to any increase. Since it is desirable that the patients be housed in the same premises in which they are fed and examined, you will have my full cooperation in the assignment of patients to your building for rental of rooms or apartments after you or your operating company advise me that such accommodations are available. However, I cannot require any patients to eat or live at this particular place. In order to avoid any accusation of discriminating against the less fortunate I would like to be assured that the structure will provide housing accommodations with equitable distribution of low, medium, and full priced rooms or cubicles.
>
> In view of the substantial amount of your proposed investment, I agree that the understandings set forth above shall be binding on both of us for a term of five years beginning May 1, 1948, with the exception that if I should ... give up my practice in Durham and move to another town ... [or] if the standards of food and service are allowed to drop below the level recommended by me, the obligations respectively undertaken by each of us shall thereupon terminate. You may be sure that I will exercise my privilege to supervise the above described services and will at all times cooperate with the owner and management in an effort to keep the service on such a satisfactory plane that the new competition after the expiration of the above mentioned five year period will be discouraged. If you agree to these terms please indicate by signing the letter ...

Filed with this is a letter dated April 16, apparently from a law firm in New Jersey, enclosing Mr. Kufferman's signed copy of "the letter as redrafted by Mr.

Cobb [business manager of Duke's Department of Medicine]." The letter continued, "If you decide to sign it, please obtain another identical copy from Mr. Cobb...." It appears that Mr. Cobb's rewrite of the proposal may not have been acceptable to Dr. Kempner, for there is no further correspondence on file regarding this plan, and it was never carried out.

In 1970, its highest point, 330 patients were enrolled in the rice diet program. They were seen daily by Dr. Kempner and his staff, and kept the rice house full. In 1952, Mrs. Smith turned her rice house operation over to Mrs. Hazel Vickers and Mrs. Aline Hogan, another practical nurse who had worked in the rice house with Mrs. Smith. In 1956, Mrs. Newton sold the rice house on Mangum Street to Ophelia Bailey (later Mrs. Ed Woody), who in 1973 sold the house with all furnishings and equipment to Mrs. Vickers. Mrs. Vickers closed down her rice house on Lamond Street and remodeled and enlarged the Mangum house sufficiently to absorb the Lamond clientele into its ongoing operation.

Along with the additional patients taking meals there came a demand for more lodging convenient to the rice house, preferably within walking distance; a number of houses in the neighborhood flourished as rooming houses. This situation unavoidably put a burden on traffic and parking in the tranquil, leafy street. When a ricer's car backing out of the Mangum house driveway hit and damaged a neighbor's fence, the neighbor complained to the city, and on September 4, 1974, Mrs. Vickers received a letter from the City of Durham's Superintendent of Inspections:

> You recall that ... I have talked with you about the current operation of the Rice House at 1111 N. Mangum Street ... centered around the fact that the magnitude of the operation and the number of people being served at this particular facility has increased substantially during the past year.... In addition to this substantial increase, it is my feeling that the character of this operation has changed considerably since the time at which this and similar facilities were established as a type of boarding and/or rooming house.

The house's food service operation, the letter pointed out, classified it among "[r]estaurants, including all eating places except drive-ins and night clubs," which facilities "are permitted in commercial and industrial zones only."

> I realize that this is an old established operation within the city and can fully appreciate the many problems attendant to relocating such a facility. However, it is my responsibility to officially notify you that the operation of the Rice House at 1111 North Mangum Street is in vio-

lation of the Zoning Ordinance and it is for this purpose that this letter is written. You are requested to take appropriate steps within a period of 90 days from this date to eliminate this violation....

When the blow fell, Dr. Kempner was abroad on his annual vacation. In his absence Mrs. Vickers contacted her lawyer, who began to marshal the defense, obtaining notarized statements from Mrs. Vickers's predecessors, Mrs. Newton and Mrs. Woody. Mrs. Newton's said, in part,

> Before I undertook this project I visited persons in the neighborhood to inquire if there would be any objections ... I went to City Hall and reviewed my plans with the authorities in charge and received proper clearance.

She went on to say—and Mrs. Vickers' statement obtained a few weeks later repeated the same assertion,

> I have seen Dr. Kempner treat some patients who were lame and became able to walk and who were blind and became able to see. We had patients from all over the world including various physicians to visit us and study our operation. While the special diet may not be comparable to a nursing home, rest home or hospital, it is a place where people do convalesce and receive special diet treatment under Dr. Kempner and his staff.
>
> While I was operating the special diet home I did not feel that the character of the neighborhood was being hurt but on the other hand I thought it was being improved. This operation is of long standing and during my ownership no one in the neighborhood complained to me of my operation but I had the feeling that they were pleased that I was there. I feel that closing up this operation would cause an undue hardship on Mrs. Vickers, a widow. Mrs. Vickers' equipment would be rendered practically useless. I have the feeling that a special use permit would be equitable and would benefit the neighborhood as a whole.

Mrs. Vickers typed up flyers for distribution in the neighborhood:

### DEATH OF THE "RICE HOUSE"?

Due to complaints from some of our neighbors, the Durham Zoning Board of Adjustments is passing on the question of whether the Rice House at the location on Mangum Street will have to go out of business because of Zoning Restrictions adopted after the Rice House began operations some 28 years ago.

With all its limitations, the Rice House has helped thousands upon thousands regain health, lose weight and return to a more normal life.

The "Ricers" have contributed hundreds of thousands of dollars to Duke University Hospital and a like amount to the economy of the City of Durham.

A hearing is scheduled before the Zoning Board of Adjustment on Tuesday, October 22nd, in the Durham City Hall (Council Chamber) at 11 a.m.

PLEASE ATTEND THE SESSION TO SHOW YOUR CONCERN!

If you care to write a letter address it to the Durham Zoning Board of Adjustment and send it to the "Rice House" attorney:

Mr. Allston Stubbs
202 Home Savings & Loan Bldg.
Durham, North Carolina

If you are willing to be a witness, please so indicate.

Hogan-Vickers.

The newspaper gave page-one coverage to the city's challenge to "the famous Rice House": "Zoning Problems Hit Durham's Rice House—Hearing Scheduled Oct. 22." [Durham Morning Herald 10/12/74]. Letters supporting the rice house arrived at the lawyer's office from Durham merchants, the YMCA, hotels and motels, and a shopping center. ["Board of Adjustments to Ponder Fate of Rice House." DMH 10/22/74] Residents from the surrounding neighborhood submitted a petition for its continuation.

When Dr. Kempner returned, he lost no time in pulling in reinforcements. On October 14, he wrote to Governor Jim Holshouser, who had himself been Kempner's patient some years before. "The Mangum Rice House is the good old Rice House in which you were lying for many months in 1957," Kempner reminded him.

It has helped Duke Hospital to extend treatment to a great number of patients who otherwise could not have been taken care of. It has been a lucky place because, fortunately, most of our patients have got rid of their diseases there and had a full and healthy life.

I cannot understand after all my patients and I have done for the City of Durham that a letter like the enclosed one from the Inspections Division should have been written. They ask me and my associates to leave our working place which we have had for 28 years by December 4th and to find within these few weeks a suitable new house, to buy it, to equip it and to move all the patients from one place to the other.

It would also be a great hardship for Mrs. Vickers, the owner, who has put all her money into remodeling the Rice House just one year ago.

There is much talk going on about bringing new industries to North Carolina. Already in 1950, there were articles like the enclosed ... How can the City Inspections Division write such a letter with reference to the place where this "industry" has been going on for 38 years....

The article referred to by Dr. Kempner, from the March 21, 1950, Durham Morning Herald, said in part,

Dr. Walter Kempner of Duke University Hospital yesterday was described as Durham's one-man industry bringing $1,800,000 here annually. In a talk before the Rotary Club, Frank Pierson, executive secretary of the Durham Chamber of Commerce, explained that the average person who comes here for the rice diet sponsored by Dr. Kempner spends $4,000 in the 110 days the diet requires.

On the same day, Dr. Kempner sent a letter to Mrs. James Semans. Born Mary Duke Biddle, she is a granddaughter of the university's founders, and indisputably Durham's First Citizen. "Dear Mrs. Semans," he wrote. "I would like to exploit you. Do you know anybody who could help with the Rice House Zoning problem which you might have read about in the newspaper? I am enclosing some papers about it."

The lawyer, Allston Stubbs, apparently even approached the Governor's office about declaring an official day in honor of Walter Kempner, but nothing came of this strategy:

Following up on our telephone conversation, I feel that it would be entirely in order for Governor Holshouser to issue a proclamation declaring Sunday, October 20 as Dr. Walter Kempner day in recognition of his outstanding service for over a period of some 38 years to persons suffering from hypertensive and vascular disease, heart, kidney and brain disease and obesity, with the rice diet.... Time is of the essence and any favorable publicity of this world renowned program by the Governor will be appreciated.... [letter October 14, 1974]

At the hearing on October 22, the Durham Board of Adjustment reversed the finding of the Inspections Division and ruled that the Mangum Street house could continue operating as a rice house. In its ruling it did strongly recom-

mend that the city's traffic division closely enforce traffic laws in the neighborhood, and that the rice patients "bend over backward so their neighbors
would be proud to have them in the neighborhood." ["Location Legal for Rice
House." DMH 10/22/74] Thus the rice house continued its robust operation on
Mangum Street for another 18 years.

Also in 1974, there was another serious attempt to persuade Dr. Kempner
to expand his facilities. Herbert Cook, a former patient from Pennsylvania,
wrote [May 1, 1974] to tell him that he and another patient, Leonard Shore,
had met with the business manager of Duke's Private Diagnostic Clinic:

> Doctor, when I visited you for the first time two years ago, I was
> only business minded—with no regard for anything else. You taught
> me an entirely new set of priorities and a philosophy of life which I
> never took time to think about prior to our meeting. One goal of
> many I would like to accomplish is to help others as you and your
> staff helped me during my treatment at Duke. Leonard has the same
> feelings and desires.
>
> In all due respect, we recognize the need of improving and ex-
> panding your program in order to reach out to more people and have
> more successful "ricers." ... We have prepared and attached a prelim-
> inary outline which substantially reflects our ideas. We estimate the cost
> of this project to run between $8 to $10 million dollars which we are
> prepared to handle. We are also prepared to spend the necessary time
> to carry this project through to the end.

The letter was accompanied by a remarkable list of the proposed facilities, comprising full clinical, laboratory and administrative space; residential space for 300 patients, including "300 rooms completely furnished and
equipped with color TV, twin double beds, private bath and sitting area";
two separate dining rooms "to eliminate boredom for the patients"; in-house
recreation space to include indoor and outdoor tennis courts, indoor and
outdoor pools, card rooms (separate for men and women), theater "for danc-
ing, movies, and nite club entertainment," hobby room, outdoor basketball
and volleyball courts, and indoor and outdoor horseshoes and shuffleboard.
The promoters took pains to make clear on page 1, however, that the clinic
was "positively *not* to have a 'Spa' image ... to the contrary, it's to be a very
disciplined situation; a 'get tough' attitude ... you can't ever come back if
you don't succeed the first time." But, like all its predecessors, this proposal
also came to nothing.

In 1976, Dr. Kempner moved his office from Duke Hospital to the Mangum
Street rice house. In that same year, Mrs. Vickers bought out her partner, Mrs.

Hogan, and subsequently brought in her niece, Billie Thomas, to help run the Mangum Street house. In time Mrs. Thomas bought out Mrs. Vickers, and eventually Mrs. Thomas's son took over and continued to run the rice house until Dr. Kempner's retirement in April 1992.

# In the Laboratory

Until 1944, Dr. Kempner's laboratory work, which was devoted almost entirely to his research on cellular physiology, took place in a corner of the two-room office assigned to him in the preclinical physiology and biochemistry area of the medical school. In these cramped quarters, he also conducted office work and, with the help of Dr. Schlayer, taught his classes, with tea prepared over the Bunsen burner and served in beakers.

With the expansion of the diet program and its influx of patients into the rice houses, a corresponding enlargement of Dr. Kempner's laboratory operations was needed. Starting in 1946, Dr. Kempner was able to expand his work space to include an excellent clinical facility, and, presumably through the intercession of Dr. Hanes, he relocated the lab to a larger space on the fourth floor of the hospital. The expansion benefited both patients and medical staff. Instead of the frequently long waits to get test results from the hospital labs, blood could be drawn right where the patients were—at bedside for inpatients, or at the rice houses—and results were available on the same day or, in cases of emergency, within a few hours. This newly enlarged laboratory space accommodated three categories of work: a continuation of cellular research, monitoring the patients on the diet, and food analysis.

The laboratory's primary activity was to oversee the patients' safety and progress by monitoring the diet's effects as well as the patients' adherence to the regimen. Because of the extreme restriction of salt in the diet, Dr. Kempner checked the serum electrolytes of each patient every two to four weeks, and more often for patients with advanced kidney disease. Where indicated, he could modify the diet to maintain internal balance. Few doctors were interested in serum electrolytes prior to Dr. Kempner's pioneering work, and so the methods available for these determinations were quite primitive. The chloride determination was a simple titration procedure, but sodium determinations were more cumbersome, involving the use of uranium to precipitate the sodium salt, which we weighed in lovely little cylindrical vessels. We procured the infinitesimal amounts of non-radioactive uranium required without difficulty from a chemical supply house. The potassium determination, which required about thirty-six hours to complete, involved reducing serum to ash at high temperatures and then dissolving the residue and forming a colored compound, which we could measure. This laborious process was complicated by the fact that potassium leaches out of glass, and so special quartz vessels were required. These sodium, potassium, and chloride determinations, absolutely necessary to maintain a safe electrolyte balance for the patients, imposed a substantial burden of work.

Between 1945 and 1947, while in medical school in nearby Chapel Hill, I worked about twenty hours a week in Dr. Kempner's laboratory measuring electrolytes in the patients' serum, urine, and blood.* I was for a short time the only person in the laboratory; later I was assisted in research projects by two Duke medical students. From 1946 to 1948, Dr. Gerald Cooper, a chemist who had spent several years in biochemical and surgical research at Duke and later obtained an MD degree, joined us as Dr. Kempner's laboratory assistant. He managed to obtain and set up a flame photometer, a new instrument that greatly facilitated electrolyte assays. In 1947, another trained chemist was added to the staff to help Dr. Ernst Peschel, who was by then in charge of Dr. Kempner's laboratory. Gradually, we were building a permanent laboratory staff. By 1951 there were 14 people working in the laboratory, including nine technicians, dishwashers and animal caretakers. One of the chemical analysis technicians was the first African-American to be hired at Duke for such an advanced position. From 1948 or 1949, the staff was racially integrated, without any problems. By 1954 the chemist had left. Over the course of the next few years the total number of techs and assistants settled at ten to twelve.

We measured sodium and chloride in the urine primarily in order to detect the patients who strayed and to let them know they could not get away with forbidden foods. Dr. Kempner sent out many letters like this to a patient (6/3/1958):

> Dear Mrs. B, As you know, you have not lost any weight in the past week and the salt figures in the urine indicate that you make too many deviations from the diet. The salt concentrations were [here he quoted sodium readings taken over some eight weeks]. I wish you would follow "the rules" more strictly. With best wishes,

The figures were also useful in pointing out to the patients the insidious presence of sodium in seemingly innocent foods.

Monitoring patients' response, both long- and short-term, to markedly reduced protein was an early concern to Dr. Kempner. Because protein is the body's primary building material, it was important to ensure that the body

---

* Blood determinations were later discontinued as irrelevant.

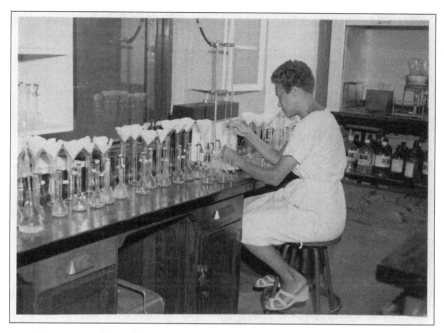

Figure 44.  A lab technician testing for chloride in rice diet patients' urine.

could maintain its vital functions without having to consume its own protein stores. Dr. Kempner initially measured blood hemoglobin and protein levels in the hospital laboratory, where these procedures were standard. His lab compared nitrogen intake and excretion to be sure that protein equilibrium was maintained. (*W Kempner 1945a; Peschel & Lohmann Peschel 1950*) He found that hemoglobin and serum protein levels stayed constant, sometimes increased, on the strict rice diet, and that the high-carbohydrate diet provided calories sufficient to spare body protein. Moreover, he ascertained that the protein in rice supplied adequate amounts of essential amino acids and was particularly easily absorbed. The fact that nephrotic children treated with the rice diet grew healthily provided additional evidence that the protein content of the rice diet was adequate.

Having recognized the connection between cholesterol and cardiovascular health as early as 1942, Dr. Kempner started ordering serum cholesterol determinations on a regular basis. Duke, however, like most of the medical establishment at that time, recognized no such connection and was still teaching its students that cholesterol levels were of no importance and in any case could not be modified. The hospital labs agreed only reluctantly to make occasional cholesterol determinations for Dr. Kempner, and otherwise restricted these determinations to patients with nephrosis and thyroid disease. In June 1944, the biochemistry department circulated a memo to the hospital staff announcing cutbacks in the number of "unnecessary" determinations, including cholesterol. In the fall of 1947, Dr. Kempner confronted the biochemistry department on this issue, as described in his letter to Dr. Stead on the occasion of Dr. Stead's eightieth birthday (October 1988):

> I had been informed by the Duke biochemistry department that they would no longer do any cholesterol determinations. A meeting was arranged at which the chairman of the biochemistry department and his associate professor were sitting on one side of the table and you, whom I had asked to help me, and myself on the other side. I argued that the patients pay for this work, and you emphasized the importance of cholesterol determinations—much better than anyone might do in 1988. The biochemists said: "We do not care. We will determine the sugar, phosphorus, calcium, and everything else, but not the cholesterol. There is no scientific basis for its importance, and it's just a waste of manpower and money."

After this rejection, Dr. Kempner asked Dr. Helen Starke, then his chief medical associate, to set up a laboratory to make the desired cholesterol determinations. (*Starke 1950*) She acquired a most unlikely lab assistant: George Skouras, president of United Artists, who was then a patient in the program, must have found time hanging heavy on his hands, because he volunteered to help out with the lab—mostly washing glassware and setting up equipment. Few labs have had such high-powered assistance. The biochemistry department continued to exhibit very little interest in cholesterol or electrolyte determinations. A biochemistry circular in 1952 stated, "Cholesterol [measurements]: can be essentially eliminated except in some thyroid diseases and overt nephrotic syndrome. Electrolyte determinations: rice diet patients can be followed by chloride alone, unless trouble develops." There was persistent lack of insight into the role of sodium and cholesterol in vascular and metabolic disease, as well as a general ignorance of food constituents. Chloride determinations were useful primarily in detecting the addition of table salt to foods, but not for detecting other common forms of sodium, such as baking soda. Thus for several years Dr. Kempner was forced to rely on his own laboratory to make these determinations, which, as he wrote Dr. Stead,

> turned out to be an advantage because of the probably greater accuracy.... But one day the associate professor [of biochemistry] asked

me to check his own cholesterol. I said, "Did you not tell me some years ago that cholesterol is of no importance in medicine?" and he answered, "I never said such a thing in all my life." Unfortunately, the figure found was rather high, above 300, and sadly enough he died not many years later, from a vascular accident. [October 1988]

As late as 1961, a biochemistry department bulletin addressed to Duke physicians gave the normal range of cholesterol as 170–340 mg per 100 cc of serum. In response to this memorandum, Dr. Kempner wrote to the department head,

> I should suggest not sending the Bulletin around in its present form. The "normal" serum cholesterol range is not 170–340, but 120–220. It might be true that a sampling of 96 "otherwise healthy" people may yield a range of the number of teeth present between 30 and 0, the average being 20. But the "normal" number of teeth does not range between 30 and 0; it is 32.

In order for us to conduct regular urine monitoring, our patients were given gallon plastic jugs and instructed to collect all their urine over a 24-hour period, two to five times a week, and deliver it to our laboratory for analysis. Sodium and chloride excretions show marked fluctuations throughout the day, so random single urine specimens do not provide reliable indicators of adherence or non-adherence. Some patients were rather horrified at the idea of making their way across town carrying a large bottle of urine.* Gym bags were a popular solution to the problem, with smaller, more discrete containers for social outings. One young diabetic patient with entrepreneurial instincts created a job for himself by making daily rounds of the rice houses and other patient residences to collect and deliver the urine specimens for a fee. With this unique occupation, he achieved his fifteen minutes of fame some years later as a contestant on the TV quiz show "What's My Line."

## The Yellow Charts

Dr. Kempner soon needed a new method of record keeping to handle all the data generated by the rapidly mounting volume of measurements. As early as 1942, he and Dr. Schlayer together designed a chart that comprehensively documented the daily blood pressure and weight readings, blood and urine find-

---

\* The wife of General Mark Clark was one of those who resisted. Dr. Ruth Peschel said to her with a smile, "I'm sure you have been called on to do more difficult things in your life."

ings, diet, and fluid intake over a four-week period, with space for medications and comments. This layout soon became known as the "yellow chart," for the paper on which it was printed. It was a kind of spreadsheet, which unfolded from an 11 × 8½ inch page to approximately 11 by 24 inches, containing 42 columns, with a small margin allowing room for brief notes on subjective findings. All the emphasis was on numerical values. These oversized charts covered with tiny numbers caused consternation among Dr. Kempner's colleagues, as they omitted the doctor's subjective evaluation and narrative summary of the patient's care—the traditional heart of the medical record.* The design of the yellow charts evolved with continued use, and their value became more evident. These yellow charts were the forerunners of the flow sheets now commonly used in hospitals, especially in intensive care units.

Two of the many tests recorded on the early charts measured the response of patients' blood pressure to sedation and to cold. Patients were sedated with a barbiturate, sodium amytal, which was then one of the accepted procedures for evaluating hypertension. Stress response to cold was measured by immersing patients' hands in ice water. Dr. Kempner quantified the effects of both procedures to ascertain whether the rice diet influenced them. When, by 1947, it became clear that this information was not of any great prognostic value and that these tests could occasionally produce dangerously low (in the case of sedation) or dangerously high (in the case of cold) blood pressures, he discontinued them.

During the early days there were also three tests of kidney function. The urea clearance test and the concentration/dilution test were soon eliminated as of no particular use; the third test, which measured the renal clearance of an injected dye (PSP), proved very effective in assessing kidney function and predicting the outcome of treatment, and so was retained. I found a strong correlation between survival and the results of the initial PSP tests in a 1955 study of 177 patients with malignant hypertension. Of 120 patients given the PSP test, 26 of 37 with a PSP excretion rate of 56% or more lived an average of five years. Only two of 13 patients with a rate of 15% or less survived one year; and none survived more than 25 months. (*Newborg & Kempner 1955*) The Peschels also contributed a clinically important measure which correlated the patients' kidney function with their ability, or lack of it, to maintain their electrolytes despite the rigidly restricted diet.

In Dr. Kempner's initial yellow charts, although there was a column for cholesterol, no provision had been made for reporting the values of serum uric

---

* In 1947, when Dr. Stead became head of Duke's Department of Medicine, he was confronted with opposition to Dr. Kempner, especially to the way he kept his records. Dr. Stead reviewed the yellow charts and pronounced them the best records he had seen.

acid, blood sugar, chest films, electrocardiograms, or eyeground photographs—not even for serum sodium and potassium. In a series of revisions to the charts, spaces for these were added, along with notes on x-ray reports and a variety of other tests.

The yellow charts must seem impossibly cumbersome to those born into the computer age, but they were, for their time, marvels of efficiency. We could capture five weeks' worth of information on a single fold-out sheet and compress a patient's progress over 10 to 40 years into a volume less than an inch and a half thick. Carrying the yellow charts from our clinic at the hospital to the rice house every day, we brought with us all the information we would have had access to in the hospital. The charts also enabled Dr. Kempner and one or more of his associates to conduct comprehensive weekly reviews of the patients' progress and problems.

Our work included research in addition to patient care. We carried out experiments using rats to study the relative role of dietary factors in cardiac and renal health. Dr. Gerald Cooper had adapted a procedure that created hypertension in rats by damaging one kidney and removing the other. He also modified an apparatus to measure rats' blood pressure. We used his procedure and apparatus for years to measure the effects of various diets on both normal and hypertensive rats. Although only a few of these studies were published, they guided us in making modifications to the rice diet. We were able to show significantly better survival in rats on low-sodium and low-protein diets. Perhaps most striking were our findings on rats with chemically induced nephrosis: eighty percent of rats placed on a sodium-free diet survived, compared to 20 percent of those whose drinking water contained sodium. (*W Kempner 1965*) In the late 1980s we began similar studies on rats with cancer, but when our laboratories had to close down in accordance with new federal regulations against private medical laboratories, these experiments were discontinued. However, there had been some indication that the rice diet, with the addition of tomato, might protect against cancer.* (An interesting rumor circulated among the ricers that in our labs we kept one rat representing each of the patients, on which we conducted experiments related to their individual cases.)

Food analysis, which we began in 1948, was the third task performed in Dr. Kempner's laboratory. Before government-mandated food labeling was estab-

---

* It is interesting to note current interest in associations between diet and cancer, Alzheimer's disease, and macular degeneration. We had noticed, over time, an unusually low incidence of these common diseases among our patient population and wondered whether our patients were genetically protected from these diseases, or whether the diet played a role.

lished in 1981, food analysis was not easily available. Despite every effort to maintain strict guidelines, patients often failed to get good results on the diet at home because they had no accurate information about the food they were eating, especially processed foods. "Silent" sodium was pervasive. They submitted samples of various products to our laboratories for analysis. A few products labeled "low sodium" turned out to be egregiously mislabeled. Even drinking water could be a source of trouble, as some natural water supplies had considerable sodium. Some domestic wines also contained too much sodium, not from the grapes themselves, it turned out, but because the wine had been stored in barrels that had been "cleaned" with a salt solution. (*Newborg 1965*) One patient who bought watermelon from a local stand found that the vendor washed his counter-top with salt water, which made its way into the fruit. Other patients found out that their coffee had been "clarified" by the addition of salt.

The enterprising wife of one long-term patient from Chicago, Mrs. Marion Kuhn, created a recipe for salt-free bread for her husband and began supplying it to friends and later sold it to other rice patients. She was scrupulous in her efforts to develop a product that met Dr. Kempner's requirements, and as she was working out the proper formula, she arranged with our laboratory to analyze each batch of bread and all the ingredients. Whenever a new supply of a particular ingredient was needed, she sent a sample of it to our laboratory to ensure that its components had not changed. Soon other bakers were marketing sodium-free bread. In addition, a number of processed food manufacturers offered to supply Dr. Kempner with sodium-free versions of their products, and the laboratory tested the samples they furnished. Other foods analyzed included so-called "low-sodium" rice-based concoctions, jams, jellies, pickles, fruits, vegetables, medications, and sauces. Many were acceptable and a boon to our dieters; others were unacceptably high in sodium and were rejected.

My work in the lab included some facets of protein metabolism, such as measuring the urine excretion of creatinine and creatine (substances related to muscle metabolism) and sulfates and phosphates (important in acid-base balance). (*W Kempner 1948a*) I had learned that creatinine excretion did not vary from day to day and in fact was so constant that it could be used to indicate whether patients' urine samples had in fact been collected correctly over a 24-hour period. With this in mind, when I detected a low creatinine value in samples from the president of a major US corporation, I confronted him, indicating that I thought his urine collection was faulty. He informed me, with mock indignation, that he had done more difficult things in his life than make urine collections. In fact, it turned out that he had done it correctly and what I had been taught was wrong: creatinine and creatine output are tied to dietary protein intake, and were thus lowered by the rice diet. He was an excellent, meticulous patient, one of our best. He lived twelve years on the diet, taking his rice diet meal along with him in a matter-of-fact way even when presiding over board meetings of hundreds of people.

An outside commission, probably from the Public Health Service, once visited the laboratory with Dr. Kempner. When he praised his laboratory staff for their accuracy, the visitors asked, "Why do you think that is?" In reply, Dr. Kempner turned to a nearby technician and asked her how many years she had been working with him. She said, "Twenty-six years." The next one said, "Twenty-five years." And so on. To Dr. Kempner, this degree of experience, loyalty, and commitment to his laboratory was explanation enough. Not only were the results completely reliable but the laboratory procedures were very well organized.

In 1987, Duke began to move some facilities into available space in the community to accommodate its continually expanding operations. As part of this expansion, our laboratory was relocated to the Duke Homestead, an old Duke family tobacco farm being used by the university as a vivarium, housing experimental animals. Although this move into an empty building on the farm at first appeared a great inconvenience, it actually worked out very well. Among its advantages were considerably more work space and available convenient parking. We were there for three years, and then in 1990 the laboratory moved back into town to rejoin Dr. Kempner's relocated clinic, in a building on Green Street about one mile from the hospital. Ours was, I believe, one of more than fifty such facilities moved off campus to accommodate Duke's growth. Shortly thereafter, responding to perceived conflict-of-interest abuses, a new federal regulation called for the closing of all physician-run laboratories to prevent doctors from ordering, and profiting from, unnecessary tests. This was a blow to Dr. Kempner, as his treatment depended on more detailed and rapid laboratory tests than the cumbersome hospital set-up could provide.

# Building the Financial Foundations

The financial structure of Dr. Kempner's program and its relationship with Duke University were complex. Following the 1929 stock market crash and the ensuing depression, many patients at Duke Hospital and elsewhere had a hard time paying for medical care, and billing collections declined. At the same time, Duke's medical staff was stretched thin to cover the rapidly expanding number of patients and had too little time for research, education, and, for that matter, rest. To address these problems, in 1931 Dr. Deryl Hart, chairman of the Department of Surgery, set up a voluntary cooperative group practice of physicians and surgeons aimed at providing a more equitable distribution of both work and revenues. The Duke Private Diagnostic Clinic (PDC), as it became known, was located in Duke Hospital but financially separate from the university. All members limited their patient care to Duke's outpatient clinics or hospital wards, without the external private practices that were customary in other hospitals. Members of the PDC no longer billed their patients directly; all fees were collected and pooled by the PDC itself. The university made several deductions from these pooled fees, and of the money remaining an amount was allocated to each physician, based on his total collections for the previous year. From this allocation approximately five percent went to a medical center research fund; the remainder went to the physician, and to his staff salaries. This closed-circuit arrangement saved doctors the costs of maintaining an external practice and relieved their offices of a good deal of administrative work. It also gave the departments of surgery and medicine some degree of financial independence.

When Frederic Hanes became chairman of the Department of Medicine in 1933, he took over this innovative financing structure. Dr. Hanes, a member of one of North Carolina's wealthiest families, never took any PDC revenue for himself. In 1937 the PDC was divided in two—Medical PDC and Surgical PDC. In that same year, Dr. Hanes's mother established the Anna H. Hanes Research Fund, which supported salaries, instruments and supplies for research and teaching, both within the Department of Medicine and in preclinical research departments, such as physiology and pharmacology, that generated no revenue of their own. Once this fund was in place, the five percent research deduction from each doctor's medical revenues was redirected to it. This percentage soon became variable, proportionate to each doctor's adjusted annual revenue. By 1946, after the usual university deductions, nearly thirty percent of Dr. Kempner's allocated money was going to the research fund, twice that of the next highest contributor. A few faculty members paid nothing. Dr. Kempner's net was about one third of the amount collected by the university. As the first physician to hold a research appointment in the Department of Medicine, Dr. Kempner was one of the few doctors to receive support from the Anna H. Hanes fund, a $10,000 annual allotment to his laboratory. This was only a small fraction of the amount he was paying into the fund.

The establishment of the first rice house in 1945 put Dr. Kempner's clinic in an ambiguous position with regard to the Medical PDC. The PDC billing structure was applied not only to Dr. Kempner's hospital and clinic patients but also to the many patients who lived in town and were treated at the rice houses. Even though Dr. Kempner saw and treated these patients outside the hospital, his program did not qualify as an external practice because these patients too were processed and billed through Duke, and the usual deductions applied to them. The rice houses themselves were owned and run independently by their proprietors, who charged Dr. Kempner's patients room and board separately. When Dr. Kempner's office scheduled new patient appointments, their names were forwarded to the PDC office, which sent them a letter with estimated fees. After their arrival and initial clinical work-up by Dr. Kempner, they were interviewed in the PDC office, where their final fees were set. Fees covered the initial clinical exam, which varied with the number and type of tests ordered, and the entry appointment with Dr. Kempner, as well as any recommended consultations with other physicians. If Dr. Kempner and the patient agreed that the patient should enroll in the rice diet program, a further weekly fee was charged to cover daily medical supervision by Dr. Kempner and his staff. This fee, at Dr. Kempner's insistence, ranged from no charge, in cases where the patient was unable to pay, to $150 per week. This charge, which was regularly reviewed and adjusted as needed by Dr. Kempner and Mr. Cobb, the PDC business manager, was unique to Dr. Kempner, as only he had a large contingent of patients living in the community and receiving treatment there. As Dr. Kempner's reputation grew, his income from the PDC, after the standard deductions and salaries for his staff, grew dramatically from $584 in 1942, to $42,683 in 1945, to $878,165 in 1971.

Dr. Kempner originally paid bonuses to his staff via the PDC, but when, in 1969 or 1970, he was told that the university was charging fifteen percent overhead simply for writing these checks, he discontinued this practice and paid the bonuses privately.

Dr. Kempner's practice quickly outgrew available facilities. He was running his program in the Davison Building of Duke South Hospital, out of two small rooms that served as both laboratory and office. Dr. Kempner discussed his growing space requirements with Dr. Hanes, his steadfast supporter in the department, and Hanes promised to help. An undated letter from Hanes says, "I think I see my way clear to getting you a series of rooms including a large laboratory. I'll talk it over on my return [from vacation]." But on March 25, 1946, Frederic Hanes died, and Dr. David T. Smith was named interim chairman. How the Department of Medicine would be run without Dr. Hanes's very strong leadership no one could predict. Dr. Kempner wrote (April 4, 1946) to one of his patients in New York, James L. Madden (1892–1972):

> I am afraid that Dr. Hanes' death may make a lot of difference in the situation here.... As you know, he invited me to Duke twelve years ago and has during all this time done everything possible to facilitate my work as teacher, physician, and scientist. I should like to feel some assurance that his successor will be equally cooperative and helpful. I wish I knew what practical step to take.... I believe you are right and that I should perhaps try to get some money for an independent research fund.... You see today I am the patient seeking expert advice, but I am very anxious to go on with my work without too much interference.

Another one of his early patients, Frank Lawrence, the president of AT&T, also took an interest in Dr. Kempner's financial affairs. In May 1946, Dr. Kempner asked him for advice about raising funds. Lawrence suggested appealing to the Rockefeller Foundation and in fact took the initiative, shortly after his visit, of approaching a friend on the Foundation board, who asked him for a letter describing Kempner's work. Lawrence asked Dr. Kempner to send him a description of "what you have been able to accomplish, and what you hope to do if you have the means to do it with." Dr. Kempner replied:

> As to the two questions ...
> 1. In more than ten years of clinical research and laboratory experimentation, I have developed a method for treating patients with kidney disease and hypertensive vascular disease with special diets, the most effective up to now being the Rice Diet.... It has been found that severe pathological conditions in hypertensive vascular disease and kidney disease which had previously been considered irreversible, such as advanced retinopathy, heart disease, and uremia, can actually be reversed.
> 2. In the future we want to do two things. First, treat patients with these diseases under the best possible conditions and with the best

methods so far available, second, continue under more favorable conditions laboratory research and clinical investigation with the purpose of improving present methods and finding new methods for the treatment of these diseases.

In reply, the Rockefeller Foundation recommended that Lawrence redirect his inquiry on Dr. Kempner's behalf to the Life Insurance Medical Research Fund, which was "especially interested in diseases of the circulatory system, [as] we have decided not to include research work in that field in our program." This group awarded Dr. Kempner his first external grant in 1947, for $10,500; this was twice renewed. One should bear in mind that, at that time, his laboratory's total annual operating budget was $12,500.

Dr. Kempner's concern about the future of the rice program after Dr. Hanes's death was well founded. His growing fame, wealth, and success, along with his lack of collegiality—he did not attend department meetings, nor did he play cards or golf or attend cocktail parties or follow sporting events—stirred resentment and jealousy among other physicians. Their coolness toward him may have been aggravated by anti-Semitism and suspicion of foreigners as well. A number of his colleagues would not have been sorry to see the last of him. When Eugene Stead was hired as Dr. Hanes's successor, Dr. David Smith recalled,

> [Medical school dean Wilburt] Davison sent Dr. Ruffin out to my house with the message that I was to fire Kempner before Stead came to Duke. I sent back the message to Davison that I would not because it would not be fair to Kempner or to Stead, who was a heart specialist himself. He could determine whether he wanted to keep Kempner or not. (*Wagner et al 1978 p 188*)

When Dr. Stead arrived at Duke in 1947, he was made aware that many in the department would be happy to see Dr. Kempner go. But Dr. Stead had a mind of his own. He made rounds with Dr. Kempner, visited his laboratory, and studied his records. He also talked with the medical residents and interns, who were very impressed with the results of Dr. Kempner's treatment. Not only did Dr. Stead not fire Dr. Kempner, he promoted him immediately from assistant to associate professor, then in 1952 to full professor, and helped him find more funding for his laboratory.

Meanwhile, there were other patients who, hoping to ensure the future of the program that had saved their lives, became actively engaged in efforts to secure backing. The man to whom Dr. Kempner had confided his concern about his future, James Madden, vice president of the Metropolitan Life Insurance in New York and a director of several high-powered organizations, played an important role in the development of the rice diet's prominence. His influence and that of John H. MacMillan (1895–1960) of Minneapolis, another well connected executive and president of Cargill, the nation's largest grain and feed company, deserve some attention here.

Mr. Madden (1892–1972) was one of the early responders to the wave of publicity generated by Dr. Kempner's address to the AMA convention in June 1944. He arrived at Duke Hospital in October 1944, referred by his doctor in New Jersey to seek rice diet treatment for an enlarged heart and high blood pressure. As none of Dr. Kempner's limited allotment of hospital beds was available at the time, he told Mr. Madden that his admission would have to wait. That evening a senior hospital administrator telephoned Dr. Kempner urging him to allow preferential treatment, but Dr. Kempner refused. The next morning, however, Dr. Kempner was amused to see Mr. Madden arriving at the hospital with a hospital administrator carrying his bags and escorting him to a suddenly available room. Once settled, the Very Important Patient asked Dr. Kempner, "Do you think very badly of me for pulling strings?" "No," Kempner replied. "With your heart I also would have pulled strings."

Once in Dr. Kempner's care, Mr. Madden followed the diet diligently and saw immediate, significant improvement in his condition. A man of strong convictions and prompt action, he lost no time in promoting the treatment among his friends and associates. These included an impressive number of the nation's business leaders, among whom hypertension and coronary artery disease were, in those days, considered a professional risk and for which there was little understanding and absolutely no treatment. In January 1945, Madden wrote to Kempner, "The President of the Phillips Petroleum Company of Oklahoma ... called [for] the name of some doctor who could take care of his Operating Vice President who has high blood pressure.... Undoubtedly your ears were burning over the nice things I told him."

In October 1945: "I have a good friend named Dr. Virgil Jordan who is President of the National Industrial Conference Board.... He is an extremely intense worker and as a result has not really been in tip-top shape for almost a year. Of course you can surmise what I am leading up to ..."

A month later: "You may hear from a Mr. Potter, who is Chairman of the Board of the Guaranty Trust Company of New York, in connection with his wife who, I understand, is having a difficult time with hypertension."

In May 1946: "I had dinner with a friend of mine, for over 30 years, the night before last and found that he has been having some blood pressure troubles.... My friend is Fred W. Nichol, Executive Vice President of the International Business Machines Corporation, New York City ... I urged him to visit a Dr. Walter Kempner at Duke University."

September 1946: "This afternoon Mr. J. Robert Rubin called upon me to learn about Dr. Kempner. [H]e is Vice-President and General Counsel of the Metro-Goldwyn-Mayer Corporation, which, as you know, is one of the outstanding movie corporations in the United States. Mr. Rubin is troubled with high blood pressure...."

October 1946: "An old friend of mine, Mr. Bruce Barton, had luncheon with me the other day and I am fearful that he is driving himself so hard that sooner or later he will have a crack-up.... As he knew how you fixed me up, he asked me quite a bit about your methods [and] suggested I get in touch with you about his going down to Duke for a general check-up.... He is President of Batten, Barton, Durstine & Osborn, which is one of the largest, if not the largest Advertising Agency in the United States."

As a self-appointed recruiting agent for Kempner's diet, Madden sent a stream of patients whose names read like a Who's Who of American industry at mid-century. Dr. Kempner's reputation thus became quickly established among wealthy and powerful people, who constituted an important part of his early patient population. Frank Lawrence was not one of Madden's direct recruits but may well have learned of the program indirectly through him. Harvey Smith of Smith-Corona, who arrived as a patient in April 1945, later presented Dr. Kempner's office with one of the first electric typewriters, an exciting innovation and a great benefit to Miss Tilley in handling Dr. Kempner's already voluminous correspondence.

It was Mr. Smith who encouraged John MacMillan to enroll in Dr. Kempner's program. MacMillan arrived in June 1946 to begin treatment for hypertension. He had dramatic success with the diet while in Dr. Kempner's care and, as a man of unusual self-discipline and determination, he also maintained the diet very well at home for years afterward. Through his grain and feed business, Mr. MacMillan had access to extensive laboratories and a good working knowledge of chemistry. Having observed in his travels that, although he maintained a strict rice diet on the road, his blood pressure and sodium levels varied from one place to another, he began conducting detailed food analyses to investigate the effects of variations in agricultural methods such as the use of fertilizers, sources of water, and processing of foods. Also, at a time when hardly anyone accepted Dr. Kempner's observation that cholesterol was an important factor in cardiovascular disease—and could be controlled by diet—MacMillan was immediately persuaded of cholesterol's relevance. It was his practice as an employer to provide his senior management with regular medical checkups. After encountering Dr. Kempner and the rice diet, he required that the examining physician share with him only one of the clinical data reported back to each employee: the serum cholesterol value.

A very bright man, Mr. MacMillan quickly grasped the principles of Dr. Kempner's program and became a fervent disciple of his work. Within a few months of entering the program, he wrote a little article to distribute to his friends and colleagues describing and explaining the rice diet in simple language. Here are some excerpts:

## THE KEMPNER DIET

*A revolutionary development which will add years to your life expectancy*

What is your blood pressure? Do you know? If not, you had better find out, as there never was a better example of a stitch in time saving nine.

Until very recently it would have done you no good to find out, as there was mighty little that medical science could do about it ... Now the chances are overwhelming that it can be corrected and all danger of a coronary thrombosis or a cerebral hemorrhage (stroke) avoided. Not only can it be corrected, but the chances are about eight out of ten that it can be done without recourse to drugs or surgery.

Just how did this come about? Well, the story behind this revolutionary development is about as dramatic a combination of genius, patience, and luck as is found in the annals of science.

.... Dr. Kempner's explanation of how and why his diet works is as follows:

A healthy pair of kidneys can stand a lot of use and abuse. They can handle salt and break down certain fats and proteins. Damaged kidney cells, however, only partially break down these substances. The half-altered remains are returned to the blood stream. They are anything but harmless and irritate the entire circulatory system, resulting in a contraction of the small arteries and capillaries. The heart must work at higher pressure to force blood through the constricted passages.

The disease is a vicious cycle, for no matter how the kidneys originally were damaged, the result is constricted passages for the blood. These in turn mean a reduction in the flow of blood to the kidneys, which in turn means further damage, which means a still greater constriction, etc. This explains the progressive nature of the disease and makes it possible to construct a fairly accurate time scale showing the life expectancy for those with the disease who go untreated.

.... It is admittedly a tough diet. It is monotonous and many persons just don't like rice ... Fortunately, most patients realize that the more conscientious they are about the diet, the quicker their recovery

and, besides this, most any sacrifice is worthwhile if one can get rid
of the awful headaches, heart pain, and other disagreeable symptoms
which go with hypertension.

Even so, Dr. Kempner's greatest single source of failure is lack of character among many of his patients. That is why he is so insistent on
their remaining directly under his eagle eye for such an extended period as the eight or ten weeks usually needed to restore blood pressure to normal, or at least to a level below the danger line.

.... Dr. Kempner himself looks on his diet as a very primitive approach to the problem. He regards it as highly probable that once we
can isolate the particular irritants which cause hypertension, we will
be able to develop an antidote, much as insulin was developed....
Only long, tedious, and expensive research can accomplish further
results. It certainly should be undertaken.

Dr. Kempner's decision, after the death of Dr. Hanes, to write James Madden for financial advice was a good one. Madden responded promptly, as-
suring Kempner that he was ready to assist however possible ("You know
that any of these contacts are yours for the asking"). He offered his somewhat
avuncular advice—from the seasoned executive to the ivory-towered scientist—on maintaining good relations with the hospital in the absence of his
champion, Dr. Hanes. The two men agreed that the time had come to seek
permanent funding from sources outside Duke Hospital, as financial allo-
cations there were inevitably bound up with shifting administrative priori-
ties and departmental politics, for which Kempner had little skill and no
inclination.

When John MacMillan, who had already urged Dr. Kempner to consider
establishing an independent research fund or foundation, joined the fund-
raising effort, he prudently approached Willis Smith, Chairman of Duke University's Board of Trustees at the time, to make sure that the university had no
objections to Dr. Kempner's receiving outside contributions. Willis Smith wrote
to Duke President R. L. Flowers (September 13, 1946) about his conversation
with MacMillan, without identifying him by name:

[MacMillan] told me that he had found Dr. Kempner to be a most
modest individual, and one who was reluctant about even having his
work mentioned, but that he personally felt that men such as himself
should take upon themselves some duty, since he felt he owed his life
entirely to Dr. Kempner's treatment.

I at once got in touch with some Minneapolis friends and have reports on him advising that he is a man who is at the head of one of

the largest businesses in the Northwest, and a businessman of great forcefulness and success ... He is apparently able to make a substantial contribution and to have others do likewise.

His tentative suggestion was that he and the group donate money to build further laboratory and hospital room facilities, and then follow it up by securing contributions from some of the life insurance companies which he has contacts with for endowing further research work. Altogether, I could see nothing whatever objectionable about that which he wished to do. On the other hand, I could see a chance to interest men of considerable means in the University, and such interest might lead to further contributions to the general work of the University or the Medical School.

In Minneapolis, MacMillan was busy pursuing his own initiatives on Dr. Kempner's behalf. Thinking on a characteristically grand scale, he was convinced that raising the amount of money required would take more than personal contributions, even from donors as prosperous as his friends and colleagues. The means and the motivation to support Dr. Kempner's groundbreaking treatment of heart disease, he felt, were best combined in the medical insurance industry, so, in September 1946, MacMillan met with Mr. O. J. Arnold, head of Northwestern Insurance Company. Also present at their meeting were medical personnel from the University of Minnesota, including a cardiologist, Dr. Aagaard, and the head of internal medicine, Dr. Cecil Watson, who was also an advisor to the Life Insurance Medical Research Foundation. Macmillan wrote to Willis Smith (September 30, 1946) that Dr. Watson

is thoroughly sold on what is being done at Duke, but stated it as a positive fact that the Medical Research Foundation would not recommend to the life insurance companies until they had repeated Dr. Kempner's results under conditions controlled by one of their own number.

MacMillan wrote on the same day to Dr. Kempner to report that the University of Minnesota had offered to replicate his studies,

with a view that this could be used as a basis for immediate action by the Life Insurance Foundation as soon as their work was far enough along. This is a very plausible point of view and there was nothing to do but concur in it. I therefore offered to pay the expenses [for Dr. Aagaard to travel to Duke for training by Dr. Kempner in administering his treatment]. Both Mr. Arnold and Dr. Watson were strongly against any talks with insurance men until such time as their Medical Foundation was prepared to get behind you and your treatment. They are also very strongly of the opinion that publicity for your work is undesirable until such time as a substantial number of doctors can be thoroughly trained in other centers to carry on your work, and in this again I must concur.

Dr. Kempner was not pleased. The proof of the efficacy of the treatment, he responded to MacMillan (October 6, 1946), already existed in more than six years' worth of published records.

If Dr. Watson cannot be convinced by these x-rays, eyeground photographs, electrocardiograms, blood pressure charts, and all the chemical data, then a few weeks' trial in Minneapolis by a new comer in this particular field can surely not convince him.

Dr. Kempner also wrote to Smith (October 12, 1946), who had sent him copies of his correspondence with MacMillan:

I am afraid you are right that the gentlemen of the University of Minnesota are anxious to divert Mr. MacMillan's interest from Duke to their own institution. I think Mr. MacMillan told you that he even wanted me to go to the Minneapolis Hospital myself.... I believe that we can [illegible] the competition of the University of Minnesota, and I hope that in spite of this delay some way will eventually be found to provide us with the facilities to do more research and to treat more patients here in Duke.

Meanwhile, MacMillan had wasted no time in dispatching Dr. Aagaard to Duke to learn from Dr. Kempner, who was restrained in his enthusiasm:

He seems to be a very nice and earnest young man.... I spent a great deal of time with him and did my best to make his visit here pleasant and profitable.... Whether Dr. Aagaard, who so far has never done any work on cellular metabolism, can learn in a short time to produce results similar to ours, without our specialized set-up and the experience of several years, remains to be seen.... If it were possible to apply our methods according to 'a few easy directions,' then funds for more facilities and further research would not be so urgently needed. I am sorry that you have gone to so much trouble and expense, but I am afraid that any contribution to this research from the insurance companies must be discounted at least for the time being. I therefore believe that I will not refuse, in the future, contributions from those persons who have a genuine interest in this treatment.

… You know how grateful I am to you for all you have done, and how much I enjoy the way you are expressing your interest in this matter. It is good to know that in spite of the skepticism of Mr. Arnold and his medical advisors your blood pressure can be as low as 128/70.

Even though Dr. Kempner effectively forestalled MacMillan's proposed plan for the University of Minnesota to set up a study to replicate his results with the rice diet, MacMillan's exploratory conversations with the medical people there apparently precipitated considerable excitement. The University, as Dr. Kempner reported to Smith, had put out feelers via MacMillan about the possibility of Dr. Kempner's moving his operation to Minnesota. Then on November 24, 1946, an article in the *New York Times* announced the opening of a large-scale and revolutionary heart study in Minneapolis ("Minneapolis Doctors to Work in Vast Laboratory—Diet and Exercise Tests on Men"):

A laboratory with 15,000 square feet of floor space and forty rooms … is being equipped by the University of Minnesota for learning how to detect heart and vascular diseases before they become serious.…

These diseases, more apparent in the United States than elsewhere, may be connected with our mode of life. That suspicion is the foundation of the Minnesota plan of study.

Dr. Ancel Keys, who heads the Minnesota plan, says that studying the cure may be the wrong approach, that it is better to learn why and how these diseases develop. All the research will be done on human beings.

The studies are to concentrate on diet and physical activity, such as exercise or lack of it. The relation of these to the emotional state will be included.

Assisting Dr. Keys is a staff of seven professors, associate professors, and assistant professors, all working full time on this project. Besides, there are fifteen full-time technical assistants.…

The article went on to discuss further the project's rationale and to outline the study plan, but no mention was made of Dr. Kempner or his work at Duke. Dr. Kempner sent Willis Smith a clipping of the article, commenting wryly,

Unfortunately, you were right in your prediction that the University of Minnesota would try to do something about this work on hypertension. I told you they had sent one of their men to me last month and, as I see from the clipping, they are already building and equipping large laboratories.… I wonder if [MacMillan] is pleased with the way his plans for helping my work are turning out.

Meanwhile John MacMillan, indefatigable, continued his crusade. He wrote Willis Smith that he planned to keep seeking funds for a full research facility, to talk with the insurance companies, to generate publicity for Dr. Kempner's program, and to invite the nation's major medical centers to send "one or more doctors for a 10-day or two-week course in Dr. Kempner's technique." Smith himself also took up the crusade, by contacting several leaders in the insurance industry to assess their interest in funding Dr. Kempner's research.

Dr. Kempner reported to Smith in October 1946 that two more of his patients had come forward to offer help in the funding campaign: J. Robert Rubin, counselor and vice president of MGM Studios, and Alvaro Garcia, president of the Tampa Cigar Factories. Regarding MacMillan's proposed training plan for visiting doctors, Dr. Kempner's enthusiasm was lukewarm at best, as he wrote to Smith: "It reminds me of certain advertisements I used to see as a boy: 'How to learn English in five easy lessons.'"

In November 1946, after he had spent the day observing Dr. Kempner's patients and laboratory and had come to his own conclusions about the value of his research, Dr. Stead—who had considerable experience with government funding agencies—urged Dr. Kempner to apply to the United States Public Health Service for grant support of his work. Dr. Kempner did so, in January 1947. In March he received notice from the Research Grant Division that his application had been denied. But things didn't end there, thanks to the influence of a rice patient's husband.

In May 1947, Helen Ewing was admitted to Dr. Kempner's service with advanced hypertensive vascular disease and a grim prognosis. When she arrived in Durham, she was unable to walk more than a few feet unaided, but under his care she made a recovery remarkable even for his patients—walking several miles daily after just a few months—and became a life-long vigorous advocate. As it happened, her husband, Oscar Ewing, was in line to become head of the Federal Security Agency, in which capacity he wielded broad authority over a number of major government agencies, including the Public Health Service and, under it, the National Institute [sic] of Health. He was elated by his wife's recovery and deeply impressed with Dr. Kempner's research. In September 1947, right after becoming the Federal Security Administrator, Ewing wrote Dr. Kempner expressing his pleasure that "the Public Health Service is supporting your work." Dr. Kempner replied that Ewing was misinformed, that in fact the Public Health Service had not approved his initial application for funding. Ewing went right to the US Surgeon General, Dr. Thomas Parran, who reported to Ewing as head of the Public Health Service. On September 17 Mr. Ewing reported to Dr. Kempner,

I have just had an extended conference with Dr. Parran and Dr. Crab-tree about your work, and I have asked them to send someone to Durham to go over the whole situation with you, because I want to be sure that the PHS is giving you all the support it can....

On October 11, Dr. Stead wrote to the research grants division of the PHS:

I am writing in regard to your inquiry concerning the work of Dr. Walter Kempner. His program has expanded rapidly, and the university has greatly increased his office and laboratory space. My own opinion remains unchanged. I believe Kempner is carrying on the most outstanding research program in his field. A grant from the Public Health Service would allow a further expansion of this program and permit a more rapid solution of the many problems on which Kempner is working.... The Cardiovascular Study Section has suggested that it send two of its members to review the work on hypertension at Duke. The Department of Medicine will be guided by this survey.

So a site visit was set up for the Public Health Service to review Dr. Kempner's work. Dr. Kempner later recalled with relish Dr. Stead's participation in the visit of the investigator, as he described in a letter to Dr. Stead in 1988, congratulating him on his eightieth birthday:

One time my application for a grant was turned down again. Mr. Oscar Ewing, the former social security administrator, interfered on my behalf, and somebody was sent from Washington to discuss the matter with me. I asked you to come to my office and to help me with this gentleman. You came, and I introduced you to each other, and I said, "Mr. X has just explained to me that my application was not clear enough, and that I should resubmit it in greater detail and stress a number of special points." I still see you sitting there without moving. All of a sudden, you looked furious, and exploded: "If you ask me, that's a big bunch of hooey! Everybody knows what Dr. Kempner has done and what he is planning to do." Mr. X responded, "Do you know what kind of committees we have in Washington to decide on these questions?" You replied, "Yes, I have been a member on all of those committees, and I know how things are done."

The investigator returned to Washington with a recommendation for approval. However, Dr. Parran, the Surgeon General, was infuriated by Ewing's pressure on him to approve the grant, considering it an unwarranted trespass on his administrative turf, and, determined that Dr. Kempner would receive no funds on his watch, he sat on the approval. But in a short while, when Dr. Parran began trying to fill several job vacancies in the various Health Institutes, Ewing seized this leverage and refused to move on the appointments until Parran approved funding for Dr. Kempner. "So he left my office in a storming rage," Ewing reported:

> As he went out, my executive assistant, Mrs. Keyes, stopped him. She said, "Dr. Parran, you're making a big mistake if you get into a fight with the Administrator ... There's a long-distance telephone, Doctor. You can clear the grant quite quickly if you want to."
>
> So, in a few days, about three or four days later, I was told that the advisory group had approved a grant for Dr. Kempner. That whole experience annoyed me so much that when Dr. Parran's term as Surgeon General expired the following May, I did not recommend him for reappointment. (*http://www.trumanlibrary.org/oralhist/ewing3.htm*)

In 1948, Ewing addressed the Senate Committee on Labor and Public Welfare in support of a bill allocating funds "to provide for research and control relating to diseases of the heart and circulation," which up to this time had not been a high priority for government funding. Directing the committee's attention especially to cardiovascular research like Dr. Kempner's, Ewing devoted more than a third of his speech to his wife's treatment and recovery on the rice diet. The Senate passed the bill, which I believe was the first major governmental funding of cardiovascular research, and over the next fourteen years, Kempner received annual grants totaling more than $570,000 from the Public Health Service. Ewing paid for his tactics, though, earning some highly critical press attention for his use of pressure politics in the direction of public funds. (*Alexander & Slevin 1950*)

Dr. Kempner's financial interests were not restricted to obtaining support for his work. Through excellent advice from his financially sophisticated patients, combined with good luck, he acquired considerable means of his own. In 1944, thanks to the addition of private patients and the early response to the AMA talk in Chicago, he found himself for the first time with extra personal income. He consulted Dr. Hanes about what to do with the surplus cash. Dr. Hanes advised him to buy R. J. Reynolds stock. "How do I buy stock?" Dr. Kempner asked. Dr. Hanes told him to give him the money and he would get the stock for him. Then in 1945 and 1946, on the advice of patients who were senior officers in these companies, he bought shares in AT&T, Anaconda, Eastman Kodak, and Dupont.

Dr. Kempner used to say, "I get everything good and everything bad from my patients," and this applied most strikingly to his portfolio. Sometime between 1946 and 1948 Dr. Kempner made his two luckiest purchases. One day when he was talking with his patient Fred Nichol, vice president of IBM, Mr. Nichol said to him, "Dr. Kempner, have I not always been a good patient, following your instructions without question?" Dr. Kempner agreed that that was the case. "Well then," said Mr. Nichol, "Now I have some instructions for you." And what might they be, Dr. Kempner asked. "I can tell you in just three little letters," Mr. Nichol replied. "IBM." "What do they do?" asked Dr. Kempner. "Did I ask you any questions?" Mr. Nichol replied.

Another patient, Robert Rubin, chairman of Metro-Goldwyn-Mayer, recommended MGM stock to Dr. Kempner as a good investment. One of the friends with whom Dr. Kempner discussed this possibility was dubious, fearing that television, a newly emerging phenomenon, might catch on and eclipse the popularity of movies. Fortunately, Dr. Kempner decided to go ahead with the investment, and the stock became profitable indeed.

Duke University benefited from the continuing success of Dr. Kempner's diet program. As Dr. Kempner's renown grew, so did his contribution to the university. Between 1947 and 1970, Dr. Kempner contributed from his patient revenues $3,100,875 to the Anna Hanes Research Fund, $1,186,957 to the building fund, and at least $600,000 for administration. The medical center also received another $2,200,000 ($100,000 per year) in these years for the chemistry, radiology and cardiology departments, in the form of patient charges for tests and consultations done on his patients.

Two important changes occurred in the seventies. In 1972, when he reached the mandatory retirement age of 69, Dr. Kempner became emeritus faculty. While he continued to have his office in Duke Hospital and full responsibility for patient treatment, I became the physician of record for all transactions involving the Private Diagnostic Clinic. On the rare occasions when a patient needed to be hospitalized, I was the admitting physician. In 1976, following a complaint by one of the rice diet patients that Dr. Kempner had imposed inappropriate disciplinary measures, he lost his office space in Duke Hospital. With remarkable efficiency and lack of fuss, he transferred his own office to a room in the Mangum Street rice house, where he continued to run the program while his staff remained in the hospital dealing with patients as before. These changes had no effect on the financial health of his practice. Between 1977 and 1987 our gross billings totaled $15,673,000, of which a large proportion went to Duke through the various assessments.

Generous as these revenues were, they did not cover the expenses of his extensive research projects. A separate research fund was set up for Dr. Kempner within the Department of Medicine, solely to support his laboratory. In addition to the annual disbursements from the United States Public Health

Service and the Anna H. Hanes Research Fund, the work was also supported by contributions from the Walter Kempner Foundation. By 1992, when the laboratory was closed, Foundation contributions alone totaled $1,905,028. After the mid-seventies, this source was still not quite sufficient to cover Dr. Kempner's laboratory expenses, so patients began to be charged for some procedures previously included in their medical fees.

Because finances and billings were handled by the PDC staff, Dr. Kempner initially did not give a great deal of attention to financial matters. The first time he requested a raise for his secretary, Mr. Cobb in the PDC office surprised him by saying, "That's fine. You are paying her with your own money, anyhow." Later, when Dr. Kempner wished to give her an additional raise, the university administration did object, as it put her salary out of line with other secretaries. At that point Dr. Stead intervened, pointing out that Dr. Kempner had brought millions of dollars to Duke, "and if he thinks his secretary is worth more I don't see why she can't get it." Her title was changed to Administrative Assistant, which was in any case more consistent with her responsibilities, and she got the raise.

Dr. Kempner was always very generous to his staff, friends and colleagues, and to causes he believed in, and this generosity was partly possible because of his good fortune in the stock market. I remember one afternoon, probably in the 1950s, when Miss Tilley and I, both quite uninitiated in financial matters, were thrilled to call, on separate telephones in the same house, two brokers to place orders for twenty shares each of IBM on behalf of Mrs. Glaser and, I believe, Dr. Gaffron. Like Miss Tilley, I also was paid an exceptionally good salary compared to Duke standards. When Dr. Kempner arranged jobs at Duke for Mercedes Gaffron and Christa von Roebel so that they could stay in the United States, he gave Duke the money from his own resources to finance their salaries, which together were approximately $12,000 annually. Between 1948 and 1964, his total contribution for this purpose was $217,164.

Dr. Kempner was well aware of his value to Duke. The PDC business manager, Mr. Cobb, once wrote Dr. Kempner, on vacation in Europe, to inquire whether, having achieved emeritus status, he planned to continue his practice and to maintain his connection with Duke. Dr. Kempner sent Mr. Cobb a postcard bearing a picture of a goose, with the following note:

> *Dear Mr. Cobb, this postcard begs*
> *you to feel fine and fit.*
> *The goose that lays the golden eggs*
> *does not yet plan to quit.*

At the same time in the 1940s and 1950s that Dr. Kempner began to establish a base of public funding, a core group of Dr. Kempner's financially savvy and well-heeled patients—MacMillan, Madden, Rubin, Garcia, and Lawrence—persisted with efforts to secure the financial future of the rice program and to create an independent research and clinical facility. They presented various proposals to Dr. Kempner, who was glad to have their help, but pointed out that his need was not for a free-standing facility but for funding to guarantee his program's continuation. Thus arose the idea of the Walter Kempner Foundation.

In December 1948 MacMillan wrote Dr. Kempner asking for "the list of men you would like to have set up the Kempner Foundation for you, and ... a date on which you would like to have them in Durham. You have had delay enough, let's get going!" Kempner responded with a list of seven men: John MacMillan, James Madden, Robert Rubin, and Fred Nichol, who were already actively at work on Dr. Kempner's behalf; along with Donald Nelson, John H. Scatterty, and Thomas R. Mullen.

Nelson, formerly chief executive officer of Sears, Roebuck & Co., served as Acting Director of Procurement for the United States Treasury and then chairman of the War Production Board during World War II. After the war, he retired to California where he served as chairman of the board of the Electronic Chemical Corporation and president of Consolidated Caribou Silver Mines. John Scatterty was a cotton merchant who was an active officer of the New Orleans Cotton Exchange and the New York Cotton Exchange. Thomas Mullen, a steel industrialist from Brooklyn, New York, became president of the Lehigh Structural Steel Company in 1944. He was also a member of the Duke University Development Campaign. Fred Nichol, the seventh name on Kempner's list, did not become a founding trustee of the Foundation, for reasons I do not know. Learning that Nichol was in line for the presidency of IBM, Dr. Kempner had persuaded him to decline the promotion in the interest of his health. Mr. Nichol may thus have felt that any additional obligations were to be avoided. In his stead, George Skouras was named. Skouras, who made his fortune in the motion picture industry, had served overseas with the Office of Strategic Services in World War II. Hollis Edens, who became the third president of Duke University in March 1949, was made an *ex officio* member of the board. Walter Kempner himself was the ninth trustee.

The articles of incorporation were drawn up in December 1949, with the assistance of Willis Smith and his law firm, and it was Smith who, in March 1950, obtained the foundation's tax-exempt status. According to the articles, the object of the corporation was

to encourage, promote, provide for, initiate, assist, or conduct, research, experimental work, teaching, instruction, publication and dissemination of knowledge, and the diagnosis, care and treatment of patients (including those whose funds are inadequate)—all in the promotion of medical science in general, and, in particular (without limiting the generality of the foregoing words), in the following fields:

(1) The particular aspects of portions of the general subjects of Internal Medicine and Geriatrics in which Dr. Walter Kempner (presently, Associate Professor of Medicine, Duke University, and now residing in Durham, North Carolina) is now, or later may be, especially active; and

(2) the general subjects of Internal Medicine and Geriatrics.

In July 1950, the Foundation distributed the first issue of its Bulletin to Dr. Kempner's patients. The Bulletin outlined the Foundation's objectives, through excerpts from the articles and a letter from its president, John MacMillan. It also provided brief biographies of its trustees and summarized Dr. Kempner's research leading to the rice diet and the results of its application. The Bulletin's editor, Katherine Ormston, addressed its recipients:

> We are happy to send out to Dr. Kempner's hundreds of patients this first issue of the Bulletin of the Walter Kempner Foundation as an announcement that the Foundation is an accomplished fact....
>
> In this first issue of the Bulletin we have tried to indicate specifically the purposes of the Foundation and the scientific objectives of Dr. Kempner's work. In planning future issues, we want the help of the readers of this first one, and shall welcome suggestions....
>
> We feel, too, that the Bulletin may serve as a clearing house for practical information about meeting the daily problems of living on the rice diet or a "modified diet." ... Many of you have found ways to handle these problems. ... The next issue of the Bulletin is planned for next autumn.

Katherine Ormston, who edited the Bulletin from its inception through 1982, contributed valuable assistance to Dr. Kempner as a sort of patient educator, overseeing orientation on arrival and, particularly, preparing patients to maintain their healthy regime after leaving the clinic. Before she came to Dr. Kempner in February 1948 for treatment she had worked for some years as an assistant to Mary Lasker, the New York philanthropist who was a powerful force in shaping the direction of medical research, especially in heart disease. This experience also made Miss Ormston a valuable member of Dr. Kempner's team. Following its initial publication, the Bulletin continued to appear at a slowly decelerating rate: two issues in 1951, then annually until 1956; then biannually until 1962; thereafter, only three more issues appeared,

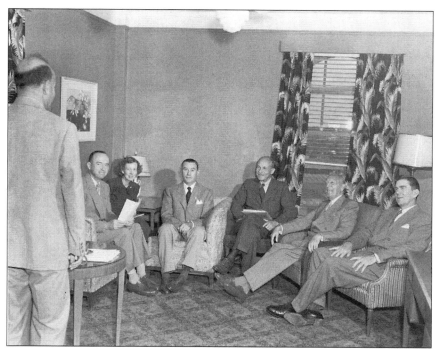

Figure 45. Members of the Walter Kempner Foundation at a meeting in Durham, October 1950. L–R: Kempner (back to camera), Cary C. Cole, Katherine Ormston, Thomas R. Mullen, John H. MacMillan, unidentified man, Hollis Edens.

in 1972, 1982, and 1993. It published excerpts from Dr. Kempner's scientific papers, paired with a simpler version for nonscientists. As time passed, the Bulletin provided case histories of interesting patients along with follow-up information on some patients as it became available. Both patients and staff contributed traveling and cooking tips. Mrs. Oscar Ewing wrote a particularly animated account of her adventures in maintaining her diet on a state trip through Europe with her husband. The President's Page frequently solicited contributions and reported on the status of funding.

From Dr. Kempner's point of view, the Foundation was a success: it attracted enough money to support his research and free him from the burden of constant applications for grants. To the men who created it, however, it did not meet with a response on the scale they had envisioned; they never quite abandoned their hope of a large, independent research facility. In any case, Dr. Kempner, single-minded in his focus on the work itself, had no interest in the distractions of administering such a facility. He knew that what he was doing worked, and he desired only to keep doing it.

Continued dependence on government or corporate grants would require that external studies replicate his results and, further, that he enter into a contractual commitment to specified research objectives. With regard to the first, Dr. Kempner had good reason—based on the many attempts around the world to duplicate his diet—to doubt that his level of success could be achieved outside his own very specialized and strict environment. The validity of his methods, he felt, was already uncontestably documented by his own meticulous patient records.

As for specifying his anticipated research results, Dr. Kempner found this a misguided request. Narrow predictions, he felt, were unrealistic and restricting; the research itself created its own dramatic signposts: neither a decrease in heart size nor the reversal of eye damage had been anticipated when he began the rice diet treatment. In an undated draft memo, he made his case somewhat plaintively but with his usual eloquence:

> I have been asked to let the [Duke Hospital] Planning Committee know what I would like. When I came here more than 30 years ago, I was asked a similar question.... I had not the foggiest idea what I was planning to do but I wanted facilities to play around with. Years later when I published my first Duke paper, "Chemical Nature of the Oxygen-Transferring Ferment of Respiration in Plants," Dr. Hanes said it is a very nice and interesting paper but wouldn't it be better if you would do something of more clinical interest. This paper was followed by quite a number of papers of an equally technical nature and with not much more relation to clinical problems.
>
> Many years later when the results of the rice diet had made it famous ... an expert was sent by the US Public Health Service to discuss my plans and the allocation of $100,000 to me. Again I was asked, what are you planning to do, and again my answer was that my plans were unprecise and vague and that actually I had no plan. I was told that there were many investigators and research experts in biochemistry, physiology, pathology, chemistry, etc., and that all of them had quite definite plans.
>
> Now I am being asked this question for the third time and I would like to say [that] so far all my findings and results have come accidentally and not as the result of my planning. All I want to do is continue to play around in the fields of internal medicine, which I also think have something to do with getting people well.

The Foundation enjoyed sound fiscal health for many years, owing primarily to a combination of high interest rates and very sound investment choices.

Its direct expenses were minimal, consisting primarily of the Bulletin, a modest salary for Katherine Ormston, who served as both editor and secretary, and the annual Christmas card. It maintained itself until the late 1980s, when, as Dr. Kempner's laboratory expenses continued to increase, contributions to the Foundation did not. The program and the Foundation both suffered several setbacks during these years, including the death in 1988 of Charlotte Tilley, Dr. Kempner's retirement in 1992, and an infamous lawsuit brought against him by a patient in 1993. The independent laboratory closed down in the early nineties. By 1994, with only $25,000 of its funds remaining, Dr. Kempner decided to dissolve the Foundation. This decision was approved by the Trustees at their annual meeting in November 1994, and in early 1995 the balance of funds was transferred to the Anna H. Hanes Research Fund (by then renamed the Duke Medical Research Fund). On July 14, 1995, Dr. Kempner sent Duke University president Nannerl Keohane a copy of a letter he had received from a former rice patient offering to donate $3,000,000 to the Foundation. "I pondered about this offer," Dr. Kempner wrote President Keohane, "but considering the behavior of some members of the University when a not very reliable former patient started a lawsuit against me, I decided to refuse this offer and to dissolve the Foundation." Dr. Kempner suggested to the prospective donor that he give the three million dollars to the Duke Medical Research Fund instead, but the man soon died, and, as Dr. Kempner reported to Keohane—not, I would guess, without a small degree of satisfaction—"He had not yet changed his Will, so Duke seems to lose the $3,000,000. Perhaps one of your associates might study this case."

# The Gadfly

The original rice diet as Walter Kempner developed and implemented it scarcely exists now except as a landmark chapter in the history of metabolic and vascular diseases. A number of later researchers, influenced by his work, wrote up their own versions of low-salt, or low-fat, or protein-restricted diets in the treatment of these diseases; Dr. Kempner referred to those diets as "diluted Kempner." He produced no book of his own about the rice diet, although he certainly had every opportunity. He received the first of many book proposals in 1948, from a former patient to whom he responded, "It will, I am afraid, really be impossible for me to agree at least at present to any of your plans for a popular book on the Rice Diet." The publishing house of W. B. Saunders asked him to become a contributing editor to a new book, *Current Therapy*, but this request also met with no success. To an invitation from publisher Frederick Fell to write up his diet in a book, he responded, "I hate to give the 'green light' because I am afraid you might talk me into doing something I have been anxious to avoid on several occasions in the past 20 years." (December 15, 1962) Dr. Kempner's repeatedly expressed conviction was that, given both the rigor demanded in its application and the considerable risks of its misapplication, any sort of "cook book" popularization of the rice diet would be irresponsible and doomed to failure.

He did occasionally seem to be tempted. In 1959, when Bernard Geis Associates was first emerging as a new and aggressive publisher of trade nonfiction, Mr. Geis wrote to propose a book. Dr. Kempner's reply was, as usual, courteous but not encouraging. Geis was not a man to be put off easily, and his letters of interest continued to arrive. In October 1960, Dr. Kempner wrote, "As to the book, I will not write it now, but I would say that it is still within the realm of possibilities." He then seized the initiative: "Please let me know sometime what your own height, weight, blood pressure and cholesterol figures are." Geis responded, "I trust you will ring a bell or sound some other appropriate signal when you are ready to talk turkey ... Naturally I'm intrigued enough to supply the vital statistics you request...." He listed the requested information, then concluded, "Now the question is: Do I need a doctor or do you need an editor—or both?" Dr. Kempner replied,

> Maybe the most useful thing that might result from our correspondence
> would be that I might get hold of you some day, put you through our

big clinical machine and find out what actually should be done in a practical way in your case.

You could make a trip here under the pretext to convince an unwilling author to write a book and in reality it may turn out that you could add some rather nice years to your life. I could then flatter myself that saving one person from falling out of a window will be appreciated in heaven more than writing 12 chapters about the ways to save mankind.

"I would have to be seven kinds of fool not to avail myself of your suggestion," Geis fired back. "I can make it any time from tomorrow on. Too bad we didn't plan this in time for the Georgia Tech game." He did come to Durham for an examination, and while here he got so far as to hammer out a draft contract with Dr. Kempner. In 1964 he was still pressing to conclude an agreement, but Dr. Kempner continued to parry Geis's inquiries with questions about his health. Geis, exasperated but still good humored, responded (April 28, 1964),

At least, you are consistent. Every time I ask you to get to work on that book of yours, you counter by inquiring about the state of my health. I'm very pleased about your concern and interest, but I wonder if it wouldn't be possible to evolve some arrangement whereby you could write a book and I could still maintain my health simultaneously.

On the subject of the book, is there any chance of getting started on this in the near future? If you are averse to signing a contract at this time, you could at least begin writing and then we could see how the ms develops. It would seem to me that almost anything you put down on paper on the subject of your personal and professional experiences, along with your recommendation for a long and healthy life, would be of interest. Start writing now and let me see the initial pages.

Geis's determination was no match for Dr. Kempner's, however, and neither that book nor any other was ever written by Dr. Kempner. Implementation of the genuine rice diet, as Dr. Kempner designed it, was confined almost entirely to his own clinic at Duke and the limited number of patients who could be treated there.

The economic impact of the thousands of patients coming to Durham for treatment was naturally of great interest to the city of Durham as well as to Duke Medical Center, where other diet-based programs have emerged over the years, some focused on cardiovascular health and others frankly dedicated to weight loss. In 1968 Dr. Richard Stuelke, a physician in private practice, came from Iowa to enroll in the rice diet. After moving to Durham and losing 100 pounds, he was hired in 1972 to head the Dietary Rehabilitation Clinic

(DRC), a new weight-loss program at Duke, in partnership with Dr. Gerard Musante, a clinical psychologist. This program was an outgrowth of a diet educational service developed by Dr. Siegfried Heyden in 1969, an alternative to the rice diet. Putting emphasis on behavior modification, it added psychological counseling and lectures to a low-fat, salt-poor diet. The DRC also offered a low-calorie diet along with lectures, counseling, and group therapy sessions focusing on the psychological roots of overeating.

In 1975 Dr. Stuelke left Duke for Durham's Watts Hospital and established his own weight-loss program, Thin for Life, in a motel in downtown Durham. Taking the approach that obesity, like alcoholism, results from addiction, this short-lived program offered intensive group experience, lectures and counseling. Dr. Musante continued to work with the program at Duke, renamed the Duke Diet and Fitness Center, until 1977. He then bought a house in downtown Durham in which he opened his own independent diet clinic, Structure House. This program closely resembled that of the DRC, but with a greater emphasis on psychological aspects of weight loss. Still in operation, Dr. Musante's facility is now housed in an expanded facility not far from Duke Medical Center.

A fifth program, the Duke University Preventive Approach to Cardiovascular Disease, was established in 1981. It can be counted among the proliferation of diet programs in Durham in the 1970s and 1980s, although its focus was largely on cardiac rehabilitation through physical fitness.

Thus, by the early 1980s, as home to four different diet programs attracting patients from around the country and abroad, the city of Durham had gained a reputation as the "Diet Capital of the World." The patients who enrolled in these programs, none of which was inexpensive, tended to be fairly well off, and in the weeks or months that they were in residence, they poured a significant amount of money into the local economy, on housing, cars, clothes, and entertainment. (One sporting goods merchant claimed that, thanks to all the dieters on their prescribed daily walks, he sold 4,000 pedometers a year.) Durham's diet programs were estimated in 1980 to be the city's fifth largest industry. Their impact on the city's finances was not lost on the Chamber of Commerce, which—after meetings with Dr. Musante—formed a committee to develop a "strategic plan for promotion of Durham's weight-loss programs" as part of their campaign to maximize the economic benefits and promote Durham's profile as the "City of Medicine."

Dr. Kempner considered the publicity generated by this effort to be inaccurate in its characterization of the various diet programs, and he was not eager to support a promotional campaign that did not differentiate adequately among their objectives and requirements. For reasons of administrative and economic efficiency, Duke meanwhile sought to merge its Medical Center-related programs into a single entity in the Diet and Fitness Center. Considerable pressure was exerted to bring Dr. Kempner's rice diet into the program, where it would share cooking and dining facilities with the other regimens. This would never have worked, for obvious reasons, and the rice diet program preserved its independence within Duke until 2002, when, under its current director, Dr. Robert Rosati, it severed all ties with Duke to become a free-standing program.

The long-term impact of Dr. Kempner's work thus includes Duke's rise from a regional teaching hospital to one of the nation's premier medical centers and Durham's continuing reputation as the "Diet Capital of the World." More fundamentally, thanks to his research, the essential roles of sodium, fat, and cholesterol in a variety of diseases—although still not given their full due—are increasingly acknowledged in current medical practice. In a symposium honoring Dr. Kempner in 1974, one of his former associates pointed out the areas where Dr. Kempner's contributions became the basis of modern therapy:

> The restriction of sodium in the treatment of hypertension and cardiovascular renal disease is today, as a consequence of Kempner's research, standard practice.... [C]urrent recommendations state that "every effort should be made by the physician to control the symptomatic, maturity-onset diabetic with diet alone ... The principles established with this [rice diet] by Kempner's work, in extreme, now have been applied, in moderation, to all these medical problems. (*Skyler 1974, p 753*)

In 1975, Dr. Kempner was one of three recipients of the Ciba Award for work in the dietary treatment of hypertension. Characteristically, he declined to take part in the awards ceremony; he was represented by Dr. Stead. Another recipient, Dr. Lewis Dahl, a physician and research scientist at the Brookhaven Institute, had also focused on the connection between sodium and hypertension, and led a successful crusade to persuade some manufacturers of baby foods to lower their salt content. When Dr. Dahl died shortly after receiving the Ciba award, Dr. Kempner telegraphed his condolences to his widow, who responded, "Your name has been well known to me ever since I met Lew in 1948 at the Rockefeller Institute, where he was busy feeding patients your famous rice diet. He always had tremendous respect and admiration for you; in fact, your name was almost a household word."

In spring of 1983 Dr. Kempner heard from friends in Germany that he had been listed to receive the *Großes Verdienstkreuz* (Great Cross of Merit) from the German government, awarded annually to about 3000 scholars, scientists and artists. The German consul in Atlanta would present the award at a ceremony in Durham or Raleigh. Dr. Kemper wrote (April 25, 1983) to the consul, Harald Nestroy, asking if an associate could simply pick up the award for him in Atlanta, as he had no wish for a public ceremony. "I have been a physician for 56 years and, without exception, during this long time I have successfully avoided any kind of public recognition or honor." The consul, who was coming to meet with Governor Jim Hunt on other matters, agreed to bring the medal to Durham. The two men had a cordial meeting, sharing an aperitif in Dr. Kempner's office in the Mangum Street rice house, where the medal informally changed hands. Dr. Kempner was pleased to show the consul a book by one of Mr. Nestroy's relatives, the Austrian playwright Johann Nestroy, which he had in his library.

Nathan Pritikin, Dean Ornish, and John McDougall have become well-known for their diet programs through their numerous publications. While none was a strict follower of the rice diet, all three were well aware of Dr. Kempner's work and acknowledged his influence, adapting and modifying some of his most basic principles in their own popular programs. They must certainly be considered allies in the fight to emphasize diet and exercise over pharmaceuticals in the treatment of many major diseases.

Pritikin, who began his investigations of diet and heart disease following World War II, was neither a doctor nor a nutritionist but a successful inventor. He pursued health studies as an avocation until his own diagnosis of myocardial ischemia spurred him to adopt a regimen of daily exercise and a strict low-fat low-cholesterol diet. The dramatic results led him to found, in January 1976, his Longevity Research Institute in California. He wrote Dr. Kempner in August that year, "You are probably not familiar with our work, but we have been following yours since 1950 … Since we consider your work so close to ours, we are inviting you to attend our [first annual] meeting. All expenses … will be paid by us." Dr. Kempner declined this invitation and subsequent ones. "Our diet very much follows your original rice and fruit recommendations," Pritikin wrote in 1977, with a request for permission to reproduce some of Dr. Kempner's photos in conjunction with a discussion of his research and dietary guidelines. "This," said Pritikin, "would be a great help to us in overcoming enthusiasm for the present reducing programs such as the 100% protein, the Atkins, and the Stillman diets.... It is our feeling that most of the physicians we have talked with are not familiar with the details of your work, and we would like to give them opportunity of learning about it."

Pritikin's institute and his research foundation have been very successful, under his direction and subsequently that of his son, and have generated numerous best-selling books. Despite his contributions there are of course many differences between his regime and the one Dr. Kempner introduced and enforced. Whereas Dr. Kempner felt that patients should stay till they had normalized their medical problems, Pritikin accepted patients for 26 or even only 13 days. In contrast to Dr. Kempner's meticulous documentation of results,

Pritikin's was mainly anecdotal. It is true, however, that many persons were stimulated by the Pritikin institute and publications to take a serious approach to their health problems stressing weight loss, dietary modification and exercise. Unfortunately, there is now scarce mention of Dr. Kempner's work as an important basis for the "Pritikin Principle."

Dean Ornish, a clinical professor of medicine at the University of California in San Francisco, is founder of the Preventive Medicine Research Institute and author of numerous books and articles on his approach to the control of coronary artery disease through meditation, smoking cessation, low-fat vegetarian diet, and regular exercise. In a randomized controlled trial known as the Lifestyle Heart Trial (*Ornish 1990*), which recruited test subjects with preexisting coronary artery disease, Dr. Ornish and his colleagues demonstrated that his regimen could not only stop the progression of disease but actually reverse it. Whereas Dr. Kempner's evidence of healing in the coronary arteries themselves was inferential (absence of angina, decreased heart size, improved exercise tolerance), Dr. Ornish produced graphic demonstration, through PET scans of the arteries before and after treatment, of decreased plaque. Writing in the American Journal of Cardiology, Ornish said,

> We can reclaim our time-honored roles of being physicians and healers by encouraging and supporting our patients as they wrestle with the difficult challenges inherent in major diet and lifestyle change rather than merely being technicians who are following algorithms that tell us which pills to dispense and at what dosage. (*Ornish 2002 p 1289*)

Dr. John A. McDougall, a California physician and nutrition expert, is another advocate of lifestyle medicine. Founding director of a residential treatment center and author of a number of popular books, he has, since the 1980s, promoted treatment of many of the common ailments of our affluent society through a vegetarian, reduced-salt, low-fat, high-fiber, high-carbohydrate diet combined with exercise.

Having been demonstrated by Dr. Kempner and then by others as the most rational, thorough, and powerful treatment of most vascular, heart and kidney diseases, why is it that these fundamental principles of healthy living—a low-salt, low-fat, low-protein diet; regular exercise; stress reduction—have not dominated medical care from the mid-twentieth century on? Because the dietary treatment of disease was on a collision course with an overwhelming counterforce: the Drug Age. Once the rice diet had established that hypertensive vascular disease and arteriosclerosis, far from being the inescapable accompaniments to old age, were *not only treatable but reversible*, the drug industry rushed to develop pharmaceutical means of achieving the benefits of diet therapy without the burden of dieting. When Dr. Kempner's was the only successful treatment available, patients had to choose between a long, boring diet and likely death. Subsequently, developing drug therapies began to be aggressively marketed to doctors and patients alike as an apparently effortless shortcut to restore health. For example, the widespread use of diuretics, a mainstay of treatment for hypertension, was and remains a popular alternative to a low-sodium diet.

But it has not been adequately acknowledged that this and other such pharmaceutical approaches only suppress symptoms, while the underlying disease process continues. When a patient once protested to Dr. Kempner that he couldn't understand why he had to endure the rice diet when he could take a pill and produce the same results, Dr. Kempner replied, "If you should find a heap of manure on your living room floor, I do not recommend that you go buy some Air-Wick and perfume. I recommend that you get a bucket and shovel and a strong scrubbing brush. Then, when your living room floor is clean again, why, you may certainly apply some Air-Wick if you wish." Another patient, who had complained because Dr. Kempner refused to give him medication for his cholesterol, told Dr. Kempner sadly that his son's application to Yale had been denied. "Well," said Dr. Kempner, "Perhaps you should give him a pill."

In 1954 he wrote to Mary Lasker [10/16/54]:

> You were inquiring as to my feelings about the use of drugs in the treatment of Hypertensive Vascular Disease. My answer is that many of these drugs can be very useful if properly employed and used in conjunction with intensive dietary treatment. However, the real difficulty is that Hypertensive Vascular Disease with all its possible complications—heart disease, kidney disease, stroke, blindness—is still treated very casually, a striking contrast to the attitude toward cancer.
>
> Since patients, physicians and the chemical industry prefer the taking, prescribing, and selling of drugs to a treatment inconvenient to patient and physician and of no benefit to the pharmaceutical industry, the mortality figures for these diseases are still rather appalling, in spite of exuberant press reports about the progress that is being made.

As early as 1955, Dr. Robert Palmer of Harvard Medical School was troubled by the growing trend he saw:

> The advent of a multitude of blood-pressure-reducing drugs has resulted in a regrettable decrease in the use of diet in general, and the rice-fruit-sugar diet in particular, in severe forms of hypertension....
> A potent urge to advertise the blood-pressure-reducing drugs is pro-

vided by the 15,000,000 Americans with hypertension, the potential
market. If not 80 or 90 percent but only half to two-thirds should use
four hypotensive tablets daily at $5 per 100, the annual value of this
market would be $500,000,000 to $750,000,000. (*Palmer 1955 p 946*)

The pharmaceutical industry's success in winning over patients and physicians as well to drug treatment came not just from the force of its marketing
but from cultural trends as well. Advertising and technology have created in our
society the expectation of instant gratification with minimal effort. The rice
diet, however, as Dr. Kempner repeatedly preached, requires commitment to a
sustained effort, for which our tolerance seems to be nearly extinct. I remember a conversation once with the chief of ophthalmology at Duke, who told me
that their standard treatment for diabetic retinopathy was to destroy damaged
blood vessels by laser treatment. This, he explained, reduced the demand for
oxygen by killing off part of the retina. This was years after Dr. Kempner had
demonstrated—with incontrovertible photographic evidence—that diet therapy, by improving the damaged blood vessels and thereby increasing the oxygen
supply, could not only halt but actually reverse the damage to the retina. In
other words, permanent damage might be entirely avoidable, if one simply had
the patience to treat the underlying condition rather than just its manifestations.

   As multiple drug therapy has become the norm in treating patients with
the multiple "disease" sequelae of modern lifestyles, it has brought its own hazards with it. We read with distressing frequency of inadequate drug trials,
under-reporting of side effects, unexpected drug interactions, and lack of oversight of drug administration. Moreover, it is too early to say what possible ill
effects will be produced by the long-term use of potent chemicals. Nine cen-
turies ago, the philosopher-physician Maimonides declared, "Any illness that
can be treated by diet alone should be treated by no other means." His words,
despite the plethora of modern drug therapies, still hold true. Drugs certainly
have their place, but they should be an adjunct to basic treatment, not the first
line of defense. This, as always, should be a healthy diet and plenty of exercise.

   A healthy diet seems to remain a remote goal for the American public at
large, however. The pernicious influence of the fast-food industry has apparently overwhelmed common sense when it comes to our patterns of consumption. Popular culture certainly does not encourage the notion of rigorous
self-discipline in pursuit of good health; food is marketed not as a source of
nutrition but as impulse gratification targeted at complex social and emotional
needs. As John McDougall said,

   The trouble with Americans today is that they want to eat every day
   all those rich and harmful foods that their grandparents never even had

the chance to eat, that their parents worked hard to buy for only very special occasions, but that they themselves can order up at the flash of a credit card and swallow without a thought for tomorrow. No wonder the body's systems break down under the load! (*McDougall 1985 p 269*)

On publication of his book, McDougall sent Dr. Kempner a copy inscribed "You are one of my heroes."

It must be allowed that Dr. Kempner himself—his cultural background, education, philosophy, and innate temperament—may also have contributed to the failure of his methods to become standard practice. I remember a passage from Goethe's play *Lila* that he particularly liked:

Any [physician] who feels about himself that he can do good must be an irritating spirit. He must not wait until he is called; he must not heed when he is driven away. He must be that which Homer praises in his heroes: he must be like the gadfly who, though shooed away, attacks over and over again from another side.

I find this a revealing insight into Dr. Kempner's attitude toward his own life and work: the evocation of the classical hero, the sense of being elected to high duty, and the conviction that no other consideration outweighed this calling. With his driving sense of mission, of personal responsibility for restoring his patients to health, Dr. Kempner felt justified in employing any means towards this goal, because he knew that it *was* possible, that their lives *could* be improved and prolonged.

In 1976, one of his patients told a nurse that Dr. Kempner had whipped her for cheating on her diet. When word reached the Duke Hospital administration Dr. Kempner was banished from the hospital premises, and this led him to move his office into the rice house. In the fall of 1993, another former patient brought suit alleging sexual misconduct by Dr. Kempner. The allegation, which he denied, stirred up a good deal of notoriety and public attention. The patient, a friend of the Hanes family, had come to Dr. Kempner in July 1970 at the request of Dr. Hanes's brother. She suffered from obesity and associated emotional and psychological complications. Because he felt a debt of gratitude to Dr. Hanes for bringing him to Duke, Dr. Kempner devoted much time and energy to her problems. He felt that his efforts met with little success. "She is in a labyrinth," he once remarked to me, "and she always takes the wrong turn." Her father, when he came to visit after she had been on the diet for some weeks, told Dr. Kempner that he had been more concerned about her drug use than her obesity. Although Dr. Kempner felt he had done little for her, her parents were apparently pleased with his treatment and surveillance, as they contributed generously to the Walter Kempner Foundation for many years.

Over time, this patient developed an increasingly obsessive emotional attachment to Dr. Kempner. She repeatedly broke the diet and, in her effort to correct her overeating, she abused illicitly obtained amphetamines and diuretics, leading on more than one occasion to life-threatening electrolyte imbalance. Finally, in 1986, he told her that he would no longer treat her. From that time on, they had no contact, although she still saw Dr. Schlayer occasionally. She continued seeking help from psychiatrists, who, according to trial testimony, encouraged her in 1993 to bring suit against Dr. Kempner and Duke Hospital for their roles in her ongoing psychological problems. The case received a great deal of sensationalist media attention when it came out in the proceedings that Dr. Kempner had whipped this patient on several occasions, and had also whipped several other patients, in an effort to motivate them. Less media attention was given to the fact that, in all instances, the patients had either themselves suggested or had consented in advance to this punishment for breaking the diet. The lawsuit was eventually settled out of court in 1998, nearly half a year after Dr. Kempner's death. Dr. Kempner, who had always prided himself on his good instinct for choosing reliable friends and associates, acknowledged his long efforts on her behalf as a tremendous error in judgment.

Dr. Kempner was as unrelentingly severe with himself as with his patients. In mid-May 1941, when Dr. Schlayer was driving Dr. Kempner to Richmond to deliver a paper, a large truck swerved into their car, injuring both of them. Dr. Kempner's injuries were serious: a fractured zygomatic bone in his right cheek and multiple fractures of his right patella. An operation successfully repaired the patella, but while he was in post-anesthesia confusion, with considerable pain in his knee, he said to the young nurse in his room, "Now, this is a test for you: you must smash this cast into a thousand pieces." The nurse fled, and when she returned with her supervisor, they found that Dr. Kempner had broken the cast open himself. The operation had to be repeated. Again it was successful (and this time the cast remained intact); the surgeons predicted, however, that he would never regain full flexion. They had overlooked their patient's resolve. With scientific precision, Dr. Kempner measured the angle to which the knee could initially be bent. Every day he directed his friends to exert more and more pressure to bend the leg further back toward the thigh, for as long as he could stand the pain. Once during his convalescence, the Duke surgeon caught him walking prematurely without his cast and asked, "Where's your cast?" "My knee is fine," Dr. Kempner replied. "It may seem fine to you," the doctor said, "but we don't want to operate on you again." Chastened, the patient went home and resumed his cast. Ten years after the accident, Dr. Kempner was pleased to send the two Richmond surgeons a picture of his fully flexed knee, along with a gift to each of a golden belt buckle.

Dr. Kempner's own assessment of himself was as "a technician and a mechanic," with no real emotional involvement. "What I have always tried to do in my experiments and with my patients," he wrote, in a letter to a friend in 1988, "was to establish mechanical, technical, numerical, quantitative facts instead of the psychic, emotional, symptomatic complaints or feelings." Regarding his practice of "the Holy Science" of medicine, he went on,

> Of course, there are approaches which are more human, more spiritual and more natural; mine is dull, dumb and more circumstantial and has been dealing mostly with figures which stemmed from experiments and test tubes. It is that of a business man or a banker, not that of a sympathetic friend or physician. One time when you are here, I would like to walk with you through the labyrinths in which I wandered with this obsession for mechanical and technical facts.

In August 1972, Dr. James Wyngaarden, Dr. Stead's successor as chairman of the Department of Medicine, wrote to Duke University president Terry Sanford to request the creation of the Walter Kempner Professorship in Medicine, in anticipation of Dr. Kempner's retirement from the Duke medical faculty:

> More than any other single individual, Dr. Kempner has made Duke Hospital an international Medical Center. While contributing to medical research, and meeting his teaching obligations, Dr. Kempner has built an extraordinary practice which has attracted large numbers of patients from all walks of life and from throughout the world … Many physicians have attempted to emulate Dr. Kempner but few have been successful. His achievements are based upon his professional competence, his charismatic and authoritative personality, and a team approach to patient care.

It is true that only Dr. Kempner's singular blend of charisma and authority made it possible for his patients to undertake and maintain the rice diet over long periods of time. Other doctors who attempted to apply his methods invariably underestimated the technical difficulties and the degree of rigor required; they eventually relaxed their efforts and could not achieve his results. His unassailable confidence and will drew to Dr. Kempner the dedicated circle of friends and staff whose complete commitment to his work was key to convincing the patients to persevere. And, despite Dr. Kempner's rather harsh assesment of himself as a mere "mechanic," his patients' devotion and his own voluminous correspondence with them reveal a physician of uncommon compassion and dedication.

Involved as he was with his research and his patients, Dr. Kempner had not much tolerance for bureaucracy and its posturing. When he received an invitation from the medical center's administrative director to attend a luncheon celebrating Duke's "Thirty-Year Club" in 1964, he sent the following response:

> It was certainly unexpected news, and a great surprise, that "the Duke University Medical Center will honor the members of its family who have served so faithfully the needs of the medical center for thirty or more years." However—though I am sure it will be an exquisite luncheon—I would rather have my thirty-year services for Duke medical center honored by a somewhat different gesture. Incidentally, may I ask how many more years would I have to work in Duke University Medical Center before the administration would see fit to provide adequate working facilities for me.

Dr. Kempner frequently expressed his praise for the "bosses" under whom he worked, however. He was aware of his indebtedness to Dr. Hanes, who had brought him to Duke, extended his appointment there, watched with growing pride his development of the rice diet, accompanied him to his historic presentations in Pinehurst and Chicago, gave him hospital privileges to treat private patients, arranged for him to have his initial extensive paper printed in the North Carolina Medical Journal, and helped him to get his North Carolina medical license. Dr. Kempner had feared that Dr. Hanes's death, in March 1946, might put his own position in jeopardy, but he found in Dr. Hanes's successor another strong supporter.

Dr. Eugene Stead and Dr. Kempner were like-minded in many ways. While an excellent physician and administrator, Dr. Stead was also stubbornly independent, a keen believer in research, and he had no more interest than Dr. Kempner in casual socializing. He supported Dr. Kempner's interests in every way, including his early struggles for funding, his requests to the hospital administration for generous raises for his staff, and his sometimes contentious dealings with the biochemistry department. The two men understood each other very well. Once when some remodeling work near Dr. Kempner's office encroached on his work space, he rushed upstairs to complain to Dr. Stead. "Come with me and look at this!" he commanded his chief. Without batting an eye, Dr. Stead allowed himself to be led to the site of the disturbance. Pointing at the mess, Dr. Kempner asked angrily, "I'm supposed to see patients *here*?" Dr. Stead looked at him calmly and replied, "Walter, you're handsome as the devil today!" Dr. Kempner laughed. "You're the best psychiatrist in the world."

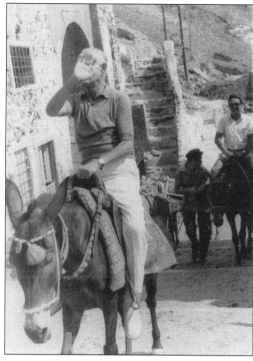

Figure 46. Walter Kempner on vacation in Santorini, ca. 1970.

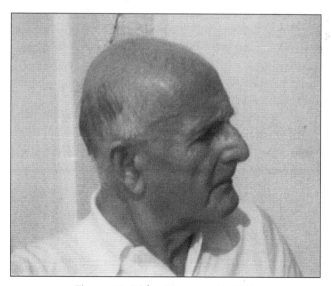

Figure 47. Walter Kempner in 1974.

After Dr. Kempner's retirement, Dr. Stead took a look back over Dr. Kempner's career for the Archives of Internal Medicine:

> It is of interest to consider why Kempner has received in this country little recognition for his tremendous achievements.
>
> He did not appeal to the scientific community. It wanted him to set up various kinds of control studies. He contended that each patient was his own control and that there were already enough studies of patients treated by other forms of therapy. He was unwilling to deny any of his patients the full benefit of what he thought was best. Moreover, he pointed to his unequivocal results on rats with experimental hypertension, nephrosis and polyarteritis.
>
> He has made many enemies because he has been honest and uncompromising and has never spent a single hour of his life, except for some scientific talks on rare occasions, in any society or even in a committee meeting.
>
> He treated all forms of vascular disease—mild, intermediate, and severe. He was not concerned about the patient's symptoms. The patient's physician at home knew that the vascular disease was in many instances not the cause of the complaining. When the patient returned home after three months of rigid therapy directed at an asymptomatic disease, the physician saw red. But in Kempner's defense, for many years he saw more destructive vascular disease than any other physician. In many instances, the disease destroyed the patient in spite of everybody's best efforts. It is little wonder that Kempner treated mild disease seriously.
>
> He believed in maximal therapy, with the rice diet being the most radical dietary restriction that he could apply. He used this diet for all patients with hypertension, heart failure, renal failure, diabetes, and obesity. He took moderate obesity as seriously as advanced diabetic retinopathy. Things are more black or white in Kempner's mind than in the minds of most other physicians. (*Stead 1974 p 757*)

Duke medical historian James Gifford speculated (in the Duke *Dialogue*, November 16, 1990) that the mistrust and even animosity that Dr. Kempner encountered in some of his Medical Center colleagues was

> in part because his results were so dramatic, in part because they contradicted established medical theories, in part because he would not support denying patients the benefits of his discoveries by placing some in control groups for comparative analysis, and perhaps because

he was a person of German nationality working during and immediately after World War II.

Perhaps if Dr. Kempner had been less uncompromising in his zeal to combat these "unnecessary" diseases, he would have encountered less resistance along the way. However, given the demands of the rice diet on both those who followed it and those who administered it, only someone with his iron-willed dedication could have achieved the successes that he did.

After World War II, as the rice diet began to be hugely successful, Dr. Kempner was in a position to give significant material support to his friends. It enabled him to employ me as a technician in 1945–47 while I was studying medicine in Chapel Hill. He was able to bring Ruth and Ernst Peschel to America and add them to his medical staff. As previously noted, he provided the funding for Dr. Gaffron's position in the Duke psychology department and for Dr. von Roebel's job in obstetrics and gynecology. His support was not confined to staff and friends but also extended to patients in financial need. For close to ten per cent of his patients, he waived his professional fees altogether.

His interests and financial aid reached beyond medicine. He also underwrote Dr. Barbara Schultz's position in the art department of the University of Chicago from 1948–65. In 1952, having heard from Judith Perlzweig that Wheaton College, in Massachusetts, was scaling down its Department of Classics, he wrote to the college president. Pointing out that "the training in Greek and Latin played a major role in my education and I have always considered this training the best foundation for all basic studies even in such fields as natural sciences and medicine," he offered to contribute $3000 a year to help keep the department operating at full strength. Judith, after taking degrees in classics from Swarthmore, Johns Hopkins, and Yale, taught for two years at Wheaton. Thanks to a stipend from Dr. Kempner, she was able, in 1952, to attend the American School of Classical Studies in Athens, where she later taught.

I do not think many people saw this side of him. He presented a reserved and wholly professional front to his patients and colleagues, and as far as they knew he was, as he himself often said, "married to medicine." (He also claimed, if anyone commented on his bachelor status, that he had been married once, "to Magog," his Great Dane.) Sometimes his patients would ask him, "What will you do when you retire?" His standard answer was that in summer he would watch the clouds, or the ocean if he was at the beach, and in winter he would sit by his fireplace, thinking of Lavoisier and oxygen, and revive the fire with his bellows when it was low.

For all his philanthropy and his belief in the potential of individuals, Dr. Kempner's life experience made him a pragmatist and a skeptic. In the end, he did not have high expectations for the intellectual or moral capacity of the general run of humanity. "After all," as he frequently commented, "sixty million people voted for Hitler."

Only on the rare occasions when he felt he was in the presence of a kindred spirit did he disclose his passionate interests and make some mutually admiring and fond connections. One bibliophile patient gave him, among other presents, an original drawing by Goethe, a rare first edition of Goethe's *Römischer Karneval*, and an early edition of Milton's *Paradise Lost*. Among patients or casual acquaintances I believe he felt that the highest pursuits and passions of the mind defied explanation and would only be debased in the attempt—it was a case of "if you need me to explain, then you wouldn't understand." He was always on the lookout for those rare individuals in whom, as Judith Perlzweig Binder said, "he saw a vital spark that he could fan into a flame."

Dr. Kempner reached the age of compulsory retirement and assumed emeritus status in 1972, and I succeeded him, nominally, as medical director of the rice diet program. That is to say, hospital billings for lab work, patient examinations, and other PDC clinical expenses now bore my signature instead of his, but Dr. Kempner continued to control all aspects of the program and to see his patients daily in the rice houses and the hospital. After he moved his own office, in 1976, from Duke Hospital to the rice house on Mangum Street, we continued to maintain a PDC office in the hospital, where Dr. Ruth Peschel and I and about seven support staff worked. Dr. Kempner's move caused no detectable interruption of the program; he maintained his accustomed energetic pace with his patients and paperwork. His correspondence with patients remained voluminous, and he still spent his summers in Europe. I joined him abroad occasionally for a week or less; as I was chiefly responsible for clinic operations in his absence, my time away was limited.

In 1992, at age 89, Dr. Kempner did finally and truly retire. By the time he stepped down, most of his colleagues and friends were gone. Mrs. Eadie died in 1981; Dr. Ruth Peschel died in December 1986, and her husband Ernst followed three days later. Professor and Mrs. Schultz died in 1984 and 1988 respectively. Mercedes Gaffron had a stroke in 1991 and died two years later. One loss that I believe contributed materially to Dr. Kempner's decision to leave the program was the death of Charlotte Tilley in 1988. Without her highly skilled and dedicated management, the rice diet's operations began to run less smoothly.

Dr. Robert Rosati, a Duke cardiologist who had worked with Dr. Kempner as a clinical associate since 1985, became director of the rice diet program. Dr. Rosati purchased property in north Durham to which he moved the rice house operations. Here he continues to run a modified version of Dr. Kempner's

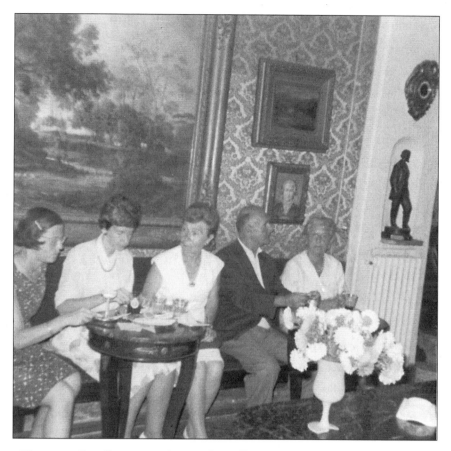

Figure 48. Traveling companions at the Caffè Greco in Rome, ca. 1962. L–R: The author, Charlotte Tilley, Clotilde Schlayer, Walter Kempner, Christa von Roebel.

original program. In 1995, Duke internist and endocrinologist Dr. Francis Neelon joined him as medical director, and in 2002, under pressure from Duke to merge the rice diet with other diet and fitness programs in the medical center, the two doctors chose instead to resign from Duke to run the rice diet program as an independent entity.

Currently, more patients are treated there for obesity, and fewer for kidney and heart diseases, hypertension, etc. Whereas Dr. Kempner tried to insist that patients remain until their disease was under optimal control, usually at least four months, many patients now come for short-term stays of two to six weeks; the diet is much more varied than the original, though still fat- and sodium-poor, with animal protein virtually eliminated. Exercise is still emphasized.

There is a great variety of classes and programs, including nutrition workshops, yoga, meditation, lectures, and cooking classes.

Because Dr. Kempner had led operations with such a strong hand, I was impressed by the degree to which he was actually able, for the most part, to walk away from the rice diet and leave it to others. For fifty-eight years he had focused his energies and his intelligence unwaveringly on one mission: to make sick people better through the application of his research findings. It is hard to imagine now, in the twenty-first century, how radical his theories were in their time, and what extraordinary effort and commitment were required to test and confirm them. This in itself is testimony to the extent of his achievements. Giving everything to his work, he achieved remarkable successes and a considerable degree of fame, and he had the satisfaction of knowing that thousands of lives had been improved and lengthened by his efforts. But he may have begun to feel that he was fighting a war that could never be fully won. Despite both professional and public knowledge of Dr. Kempner's treatment, which could by now have nearly eliminated certain diseases if fully adopted, we still have high morbidity and mortality from vascular and metabolic disorders. We seem unable to resist the allure of quick fixes.

With his new and unaccustomed leisure, Dr. Kempner was able finally to devote more time and attention to his literary and artistic interests. His library contained valuable editions of the works of Goethe and other German writers, and beginning with his trips to Greece and Italy in the 1920s he had acquired a considerable collection of antiquities. He busied himself with these and with revisiting his personal correspondence, news clippings, and scientific publications. (Miss Tilley used to complain that it was impossible to get his attention once he became engrossed in his old scientific papers.)

Dr. Schlayer, Dr. Hanna Ruestow, Dr. Kempner, and I continued to have lunch together frequently. In good weather, we often brought our lawn chairs out into the cul-de-sac on Pershing Street to listen to the Texaco opera broadcasts on Saturday afternoons. At the house of Fides Ruestow, he frequently lay in the sun on her terrace, enjoying her beautiful rose garden. He maintained his good health, mentally and physically, until the end. On September 27, 1997, he had lunch with several of us and afterward discussed his plans for a longer vacation the next summer. In late afternoon he complained of abdominal pain, and at 11:00 that night he died of a heart attack. He was cremated, and his ashes were buried in the cemetery in Locarno near the grave of Stefan George. Dr. Schlayer and Miss Ruestow both died in 2004 and are buried there as well.

# Bibliography

*Note to the Reader*: The bibliography includes all of the scientific articles by Dr. Kempner. Many of them are now available only in a two-volume collection of papers written by him and by associates working under his direction: *Scientific Publications by Walter Kempner, MD, Volume 1: Studies in Cellular Physiology* and *Volume II: Radical Dietary Treatment of Vascular and Metabolic Disorders.* Durham, NC: Gravity Press, 2002 and 2004. These two volumes are found in most medical libraries in the United States and several abroad. There are also references in the text to the Bulletin of the Walter Kempner Foundation (WKF Bull), which appeared irregularly between 1950 and 1993, fourteen issues in all. Copies of these Bulletins are held in the Library of Congress and the medical library at Duke University.

Alexander H, Slevin JR. Mr. welfare state himself. Collier's Magazine, February 4, 1950.

Allen FM, Sherill JW. The treatment of arterial hypertension. Journal of Metabolic Research 1922; 2: 429–463.

Bergmann G. Funktionelle Pathologie: Eine Klinische Sammlung [Functional Pathology: A Clinical Collection] Berlin: Verlag von Julius Springer, 1932.

Boehringer R. Briefwechsel zwischen George und Hofmannsthal. [Correspondence between George and Hofmannsthal] Berlin: Georg Bondi, 1938.

Dahl LK, Stall BG, Cotzias GC. Metabolic effects of marked sodium restriction in hypertensive patients. changes in total exchangeable sodium and potassium. Journal of Clinical Investigation 1954; 33: 1397–1406.

Dock W. The predilection of atherosclerosis for the coronary arteries. Journal of the American Medical Association 1946; 131: 875.

Fishberg AM. Hypertension and Nephritis, 4th ed. Philadelphia: Lea & Febiger, 1939.

Fishberg AM. Panel discussion on the clinical management of hypertension. Journal of the American Geriatric Society 1958; 6: 713–39.

Flipse ME, Flipse MJ. Observations in treatment of hypertension with rice-fruit diet. Southern Medical Journal 1947; 40: 721–28.

Flipse ME. Pathogenesis of coronary artery disease. Journal of the American Medical Association 1960; 172: 1130–33.

Gaffron M. Right and left in pictures. Art Quarterly 1950; 13: 312–31.

Gaffron M. Die Radierungen Rembrandts: Studien über Inhalt und Komposition. [Rembrandt's Etchings: Studies on Content and Composition] Mainz: Florian Kupferberg Verlag, 1950.

George S. Werke: Ausgabe in Zwei Bänden. München und Düsseldorf: Helmut Küpper vormals Georg Bondi, 1958.

Graffmann-Weschke K. Lydia Rabinowitsch-Kempner (1871–1935): Leben und Werk einer der führenden Persönlichkeiten der Tuberkuloseforschung am Anfang des 20. Jahrhunderts. [Life and Work of One of the Leaders in Tuberculosis Research at the Beginning of the 20th Century] 1997. Doctoral dissertation, Freie Universität, Berlin.

Grollman A, Harrison TR. Effect of rigid sodium restriction on blood pressure and survival of hypertensive rats. Proceedings of the Society for Experimental Biology and Medicine 1945; 60: 52.

Hanes FM, Kempner W. The effect of various sulfonamide drugs on pneumococcus, as determined by measuring manometrically the bacterial metabolism. Transactions of the Association of American Physicians 1941; 56: 152–64.

Hawkins WR. Eat Right—Electrolyte: A Nutritional Guide to Minerals in Our Daily Diet. New York: Prometheus Books, 2006.

Hölderlin F. Gedichte. Frankfurt am Main: Insel Verlag, 1969.

Inventory of records, Emergency Committee in Aid of Displaced Foreign Scholars (ECIADFS), 1933–45. Manuscripts and Archives Division, NY Public Library.

Kantorowicz E. The Fundamental Issue: Documents and Marginal Notes on the University of California Loyalty Oath. Berkeley, CA: Private printing, 1950.

Kantorowicz E. The King's Two Bodies. Princeton, NJ: Princeton University Press, 1957.

Kempner N. Raleghs staatstheoretische Schriften [Raleigh's Theoretical Writings Concerning the State] Leipzig: Verlag von Bernhard Tauchnitz, 1928.

Kempner RMW. Ankläger einer Epoche: Lebenserinnerungen [Prosecutor of an Era: Memoirs] Frankfurt/Main: Verlag Ullstein, 1983.

Kempner RMW. Robert Kempner 1899–1993: Ewige Wachsamkeit ist der Preis der Freiheit: Die demokratische Rechtskultur von der Weimarer Republik bis zur Gegenwart. [Eternal Vigilance is the Price of Freedom: Justice in Democracy from the Weimar Republic to the Present] Katalog zur Ausstellung. Zweite, erweiterte Auflage. Frankfurt am Main 2006.

Kempner W. Zur Kenntnis des Phlorhizindiabetes [The nature of phlorhizin diabetes]. Archiv für experimentelle Pathologie und Pharmakologie 1927; 122: 1–23.

Kempner W. Atmung im Plasma pestkranker Hühner [Respiration in the plasma of chickens with plague]. Klinische Wochenschrift 1927; 6: 2386–7.

Kempner W and Peschel E. Stoffwechsel der Entzündung [Metabolism of inflammation]. Zeitschrift für klinische Medizin 1930; 114: 439–55.

Kempner W. Wirkung von Blausäure und Kohlenoxyd auf die Buttersäuregärung [Effect of cyanide and carbon monoxide on butyric acid fermentation]. Biochemische Zeitschrift 1933; 257: 41–56.

Kempner W, Kubowitz F. Wirkung des Lichtes auf die Kohlenoxydhemmung der Buttersäuregärung [Effect of light on the inhibition of butyric acid fermentation by carbon monoxide]. Biochemische Zeitschrift 1933; 265: 245–52.

Kempner W. Metabolism of human erythroblasts. Journal of Clinical Investigation 1936; 15: 679–83.

Kempner W. Chemical nature of the oxygen-transferring ferment of respiration in plants. Plant Physiology 1936; 11: 605–13.

Kempner W. Effect of low oxygen tension upon respiration and fermentation of isolated cells. Proceedings of the Society for Experimental Biology and Medicine 1936; 35: 148–51.

Kempner W. Effect of oxygen tension on cellular metabolism. Journal of Cellular and Comparative Physiology 1937; 10: 339–63.

Kempner W. Verminderter Sauerstoffdruck in der Niere als Ursache der "reversiblen" urämischen Acidose [Anoxemia of the kidney as a cause of reversible uremic acidosis]. Klinische Wochenschrift 1938; 17: 971–8.

Kempner W. Anoxemia of the kidney as a cause of uremic acidosis. The American Journal of Physiology 1938; 123: 117–8.

Kempner W. Inhibitory effect of low oxygen tension on the deamination of amino acids in the kidney. The Journal of Biological Chemistry 1938; 124: 229–35.

Kempner W. The effects of the variations of atmospheric oxygen concentration upon the metabolism of tubercle bacteria. The American Journal of Physiology 1939; 126: 553.

Kempner W. Oxygen tension and the tubercle bacillus. The American Review of Tuberculosis 1939; 40: 157–68.

Kempner W. The role of oxygen tension in biological oxidations. Cold Spring Harbor Symposia on Quantitative Biology 1939; 7: 269–89.

Kempner W, Gaffron M. Metabolism of human myeloblasts and its sensitivity toward variations of oxygen tension. The American Journal of Physiology 1939; 126: 553.

Kempner W. The nature of leukemic blood cells as determined by their metabolism. The Journal of Clinical Investigation 1939; 18: 291–300.

Kempner W. Comment at a pathological conference involving advanced kidney disease. North Carolina Medical Journal 1943; 4: 227–8.

Kempner W. Treatment of kidney disease and hypertensive vascular disease with the rice diet. The Chicago Session. Journal of the American Medical Association. May 6, 1944

Kempner W. Treatment of kidney disease and hypertensive vascular disease with the rice diet. North Carolina Medical Journal 1944; 5: 125–33.

Kempner W. Treatment of kidney disease and hypertensive vascular disease with rice diet, II. North Carolina Medical Journal 1944; 5: 272–74.

Kempner W. Compensation of renal metabolic dysfunction: Treatment of kidney disease and hypertensive vascular disease with rice diet, III. Part 1. North Carolina Medical Journal 1945; 6: 61–87.

Kempner W. Compensation of renal metabolic dysfunction: Treatment of kidney disease and hypertensive vascular disease with rice diet, III. Part 2. North Carolina Medical Journal 1945; 6: 117–61.

Kempner W. Some effects of the rice diet treatment on kidney disease and hypertension. Bulletin of the New York Academy of Medicine 1946; 22: 358–70.

Kempner W. Treatment of cardiac failure with the rice diet. North Carolina Medical Journal 1947; 8: 128–31.

Kempner W. Treatment of hypertensive vascular disease with rice diet. The American Journal of Medicine 1948; 4: 545–77. Reprinted in the Kempner Symposium, 1974.

Kempner W, Lesesne J, Newborg B, Whicker C. Sulfate and phosphate excretion in urine of patients on rice diet. American Journal of the Medical Sciences 1948; 216: 687–8.

Kempner W, Peschel E, and Starke H. Rice diet in malignant hypertension: a case history. American Practitioner 1949; 111: 556–63.

Kempner W. Treatment of heart and kidney disease and of hypertensive and arteriosclerotic vascular disease with the rice diet. Annals of Internal Medicine 1949; 31: 821–56.

Kempner W. Treatment of heart and kidney disease and of hypertensive and arteriosclerotic vascular disease with the rice diet. Premier Congrès Mondial de Cardiologie II. Paris, France 1950; 2: 32–4. [Abstract printed in Bulletin of the Walter Kempner Foundation. 1951; 1]

Kempner W. The treatment of retinopathy in kidney disease and hypertensive and arteriosclerotic vascular disease with the rice diet. Ophthalmologia Ibero Americana 1951; 13: 1–40.

Kempner W. Tratamiento de enfermedades cardíacas y renales, retinopatías y enfermedades vasculares arterioscleróticas e hipertensivas can la dieta de arroz. Archivos Medicos de Cuba 1952; 3: 131–42.

Kempner W. Radical dietary treatment of hypertensive and arteriosclerotic vascular disease, heart and kidney disease and vascular retinopathy. General Practitioner 1954; 9: 71–93.

Kempner W. Wirkung der Reisdiät bei experimenteller Hypertonie und bei Patienten mit Herz-, Nieren- und Gefässkrankheiten [Effect of the rice diet in experimental hypertension and in patients with heart, kidney and vascular disease]. Zeitschrift für Klinische Medizin 1954; 152: 328–45.

Kempner W, Peschel E, Black-Schaffer B. Effect of diet on experimental hypertension and on the development of polyarteritis nodosa in rats. Circulation Research 1955; 3: 73–8.

Kempner W. Trattamento radicale dietico delle malattie vascolari, ipertensive ed arteriosclerotiche, di quelle cardiache e renalie delle retinopatie vascolari [Italian translation of W Kempner 1954a]. L'Ente Nationale Risi, 1957: 7–41.

Kempner W, Lohmann-Peschel R, Schlayer C. Effect of rice diet on diabetes mellitus associated with vascular disease. Postgraduate Medicine 1958; 24: 359–71.

Kempner W. Effect of salt restriction on experimental nephrosis. Journal of the American Medical Association 1965; 191: 51.

Kempner W, Newborg B, Lohmann-Peschel R, Skyler JS. Treatment of massive obesity with rice/reduction program. Archives of Internal Medicine 1975; 135: 1575–84.

Kempner W. Otto Warburg 1883–1970: thoughts upon looking at the 1983 commemorative issue of the Postal Service of West Germany in honor of his hundredth birthday. North Carolina Medical Journal 1984; 45: 25–26.

Kempner W. WKF Bulletin 1993: 6; 5–14.

Krebs HA. Über den Ablauf der Blutammoniakkurve [Concerning the blood-ammonia curve]. Hoppe-Seylers Zeitung 1933; 217: 191.

Lohmann R. Krebsstoffwechsel und Entzündung [Cancer metabolism and inflammation]. Klinische Wochenschrift 1931; 10: 1799–1802.

Lohmann R. Manometrische Untersuchungen über Stoffwechsel und Wachstum von Bakterien unter dem Einfluss von ultraviolettem Licht und unter den Bedingungen der Entzündung [Manometric studies to determine the effects of ultraviolet light and conditions of inflammation on the metabolism and growth of bacteria]. Klinische Wochenschrift 1934; 13: 1112–16.

Lohmann R. Über das Verhalten des Fermentes der Milchsäuregärung beim Glykogenzerfall [On the reaction of the enzyme of lactic acid fermentation during glycogen breakdown]. Archiv für experimentelle Pathologie und Pharmakologie 1936; 182: 239–42.

Lohmann R. Gasstoffwechsel und Glykogenzerfall [Metabolism of gases and glycogen breakdown]. Klinische Wochenschrift 1937; 16: 1682–84.

Lohmann R. Biologie der Entzündung [Biology of inflammation]. Zeitschrift für klinische Medizin 1938; 135: 316–46.

Lohmann R. Zur Wirkung des Insulins auf die Zuckerverwertung im Glykogenzerfall [The effect of insulin on sugar utilization in glycogen breakdown]. Zeitschrift für klinische Medizin 1938; 135: 505–08.

Marx O, Morwitz E. Gods and Heroes: Myths and Epics of Ancient Greece. [Translation of Schwab G. Die schönsten Sagen des klassischen Altertums: nach seinen Dichtern und Erzählern. Stuttgart: SG Liesching, 1838–40] New York: Pantheon Books, 1946.

Marx O, Morwitz E. The Works of Stefan George Rendered into English. University of North Carolina Studies in the Germanic Languages and Literatures, No. 2. Chapel Hill, NC, 1949.

McDougall JA. McDougall's Medicine: A Challenging Second Opinion. Piscataway, NJ: New Century Publishers, Inc., 1985.

Nash TP, Benedict SR. The ammonia content of the blood and its bearing on the mechanism of acid neutralization in the animal organism. Journal of Biological Chemistry 1921; 48: 463.

Nash TP, Benedict SR. Note on the ammonia content of blood. Journal of Biological Chemistry 1922; 51: 183.

Newborg B, Kempner W. Analysis of 177 cases of hypertensive vascular disease with papilledema. American Journal of Medicine 1955; 19: 33–47.

Newborg B. Pseudotumor cerebri treated by rice/reduction diet. Archives of Internal Medicine 1974; 133: 802–807.

Newborg B. Effect of weight loss on arterial oxygen pressure (pO2). Federation Proceedings 1977; 36.

Newborg B. Obesity destabilizes the system. North Carolina Medical Journal 1983; 44: 242.

Newborg B. The role of oxygen pressure in the fight against the chief killers in the first and in the last half of the 20th century. North Carolina Medical Journal 1985; 46: 47–48.

Newborg B. Disappearance of psoriatic lesions on the rice diet. North Carolina Medical Journal 1986; 47: 253–55.

Ornish D et al. Can lifestyle changes reverse coronary heart disease? The Lifestyle Heart Trial. Lancet 1990; 336: 129–33.

Ornish D. Statins and the soul of medicine. American Journal of Cardiology 2002; 89: 1286–90.

Page IH, Corcoran AC. Arterial Hypertension. Chicago: Yearbook Publishers, 1945.

Palmer R. Progress in medicine: essential hypertension: a selected review and commentary. New England Journal of Medicine 1955; 252: 940–47.

Peschel E. Stoffwechsel leukaemischer Lymphocyten [Metabolism of leukemic lymphocytes]. Klinische Wochenschrift 1930; 9: 1061–2.

Peschel E, Lohmann Peschel R. Nitrogen balance on rice diet. Journal of Clinical Investigation 1950; 29: 455–59.

Peschel E, Black-Schaffer B, Schlayer C. Potassium deficiency as cause of the so-called rheumatic heart lesions of the adaptation syndrome. Endocrinology 1951; 48: 399–407.

Peschel E, Lohmann Peschel R. Electrolyte metabolism during rice diet I: Serum electrolytes in hypertensive patients without evidence of advanced renal involvement. Archives of Internal Medicine 1952; 89: 234–39.

Peschel E, Lohmann Peschel R. Electrolyte metabolism during rice diet II: Serum electrolytes in patients with severe primary or secondary renal disease. Archives of Internal Medicine 1953; 91: 296–303.

Schlayer C. Spuren Lukans in der spanischen Dichtung. Heidelberg: Weiss'sche Universitäts-Buchhandlung 1928.

Schlayer C. Wirkung des Kohlenoxyds auf die Gärung von Tetanus- und Gasbrandbazillen [Effect of carbon monoxide on fermentation of tetanus and clostridium welchii bacteria]. Biochemische Zeitschrift 1935; 276: 460–63.

Schlayer C. The influence of oxygen tension on the respiration of pneumococci (Type I). Journal of Bacteriology 1936; 31: 181–89.

Schlayer C. Der Einfluss des Sauerstoffdrucks auf den Zellstoffwechsel und der Mechanismus der Blausäurewirkung [Influence of oxygen tension on cell metabolism and the mechanism of the cyanide effect]. Biochemische Zeitschrift 1937; 293: 94–98.

Schlayer C. Manometrische Bestimmung von Aminosäuren mit Ninhydrin im Warburg-Apparat [Manometric assay of amino acids with Ninhydrin in the Warburg apparatus]. Biochemische Zeitschrift 1938; 297: 395–97.

Schlayer C. Sauerstoffzehrung des Urins und Sauerstoffdruck der Niere [Oxygen consumption in urine and oxygen tension in the kidney]. Klinische Wochenschrift 1939; 17: 598–99.

Schlayer C. 60 Poemas de Stefan George. Düsseldorf & München: Helmut Küpper vormals Georg Bondi, 1964.

Schlayer C. Gedichte: Eine Auswahl Seit 1920 [Poems: A Collection since 1920]. Stuttgart: Klett-Cotta, 1981.

Schlayer F. Diplomat im Roten Madrid [Diplomat in Red Madrid]. Berlin: F. A. Herbig Verlagbuchhandlung, 1938.

Schlayer F. Ein Schwabe in Spanien: Erinnerungen aus der ersten Hälfte des 20. Jahrhunderts. [A Swabian in Spain: Recollections from the First Half of the 20th Century] Stuttgart: Hohenheim Verlag, 2007.

Seekamp H-J, Ockenden RC, Keilson M. Stefan George Leben und Werk: Eine Zeittafel [Stefan George Life and Work: A Timeline]. Amsterdam: Castrum Peregrini Presse, 1972.

Selye H, Stone H. Effect of the diet upon the renotropic, nephroscleriotic, cardiotropic and adrenotropic actions of crude anterior pituitary preparations. Federation Proceedings 1946; 5: 93.

Skyler J. Walter Kempner: a biographical note. Archives of Internal Medicine 1974; 133: 752–55.

Starke H. Effect of the rice diet on the serum cholesterol fractions of 154 patients with hypertensive vascular disease. American Journal of Medicine 1950; 9: 494–99.

Stead EA. Walter Kempner: A perspective. Archives of Internal Medicine 1974; 133: 756–57.

Stead EA. Kempner revisited. North Carolina Medical Journal 1983; 44: 237–40.

Valhope CN, Morwitz E, eds. Stefan George Poems. New York: Pantheon Books, Inc., 1943.

Volhard F. Die Behandlung der Nephrosklerosen, Handbuch der Inneren Medizin, 2nd ed. Bergmann and Staehelin, eds. Berlin: Julius Springer, 1931.

Wagner GS, Cebe B, Rozear MP. Eugene A. Stead, Jr.: What This Patient Needs Is a Doctor. Durham, NC: Carolina Academic Press, 1978.

Walsh LR, Poupard JA. Lydia Rabinowitsch, PhD, and the Emergence of Clinical Pathology in Late 19th-Century America. Archives of Pathology and Laboratory Medicine 1989; 113: 1303–08.

White PD. The management of hypertension. Annals of Internal Medicine 1947; 27: 740–48.

Zielke B. Die orientalische Frage im politischen Denken Europas [The oriental question in the political thinking of Europe] 1931. Doctoral dissertation, University of Heidelberg.

## Web Resources

http://www.trumanlibrary.org/oralhist/ewing3.htm.
http://www.holocaustdenialontrial.com/evidence.
http://www.fff.org/freedom/fd0403a.asp.

# List of Names

**Donald K. Adams** (born March 6, 1902, Orville, OH; died May 20, 1971, Durham, NC), a physician and psychologist, specializing in animal behavior and comparative psychology. A graduate of Harvard and Yale Universities, who also studied in Berlin and Geneva, he chaired the Department of Psychology at Duke from 1947 to 1951.

**Rosa Albagés y Gallego** (born June 27, 1867, Seville; died August 28, 1961, Torrelodones, Madrid), the mother of Clotilde and Karl Schlayer, and a contemporary of Pablo Casals at the Barcelona Conservatory, where she studied to become an opera singer. She taught voice for a few years but gave up her career to marry Felix Schlayer on March 17, 1900.

**Emmy Allard** (born September 25, 1881, Lüdinghausen, Germany; died May 7, 1953, Berlin), teacher in the girls' school attended by Nadja Kempner and Clotilde Schlayer, with whom she maintained a life-long friendship. She received a PhD in philosophy from the Friedrich-Wilhelms University in Berlin. She cared for the Kempner family grave in Lichterfelde despite Nazi prohibitions.

**George Baehr** (1887–1978), a physician who served as president and medical director of the Health Insurance Plan of Greater New York; Director of the Medical Division of the Office of Civilian Defense; and a member of the Rockefeller Institute.

**Bernard Bang** (born June 7, 1848, Sjelland, Denmark; died June 22, 1932, Copenhagen), a Danish veterinarian known for his work on tuberculosis and *Bacillus abortus*.

**Gustav von Bergmann** (born December 24, 1878, Würzburg; died September 16, 1955, Munich), a leading internist who was head of the departments of medicine at the universities of Marburg, Frankfurt am Main, and Berlin, successively. He was especially interested in gastroenterology and published the *Handbuch der inneren Medizin*.

**Judith Perlzweig Binder** (born June 2, 1921, Baltimore), an archaeologist, received her doctorate in Classics from Yale University and taught for many years at the American School of Classical Studies in Athens.

**Robert Boehringer** (born July 30, 1884, Winnenden, Germany; died August 9, 1974, Geneva), an industrialist, successively head of three major pharmaceutical concerns (Boehringer Ingelheim, Hoffmann-La Roche, Geigy) and a senior administrator of the International Red Cross between 1940 and 1946. He was George's heir and founded the Stefan George Stiftung und Archiv in Stuttgart.

**Rudolph Diels** (born December 16, 1900, Belghaus, Germany; died November 18, 1957, Katzeneinbogen, Germany), was a protégé of Hermann Goering and headed the Gestapo, which he helped found in 1933–34.

**Rosabel Coutts Eadie** (born August 7, 1894, Windsor, Ontario; died January 30, 1981, Durham, NC), worked in the Toronto laboratory of Bunting and Best, who developed the treatment of diabetes with insulin.

**Simon Flexner** (born March 25, 1863, Louisville, Kentucky; died May 2, 1946, New York), brother of Abraham Flexner, physician, professor of pathology and bacteriologist. He was the first director of the Rockefeller Institute for Medical Research and a trustee of the Rockefeller Foundation.

**Victor Frank** (born May 23, 1909, Moscow; died February 26, 1943, near Stalingrad), born Frank Mehnert. A sculptor who, after meeting George in 1924, became his close companion. He was killed in the battle of Stalingrad.

**Hans Gaffron** (born May 17, 1902, Lima, Peru; died August 19, 1979, Falmouth, MA), a biochemist particularly interested in photosynthesis. He worked in the Warburg Institute in Berlin. After coming to the US in 1938 he was on the faculty of the University of California's Hopkins Marine Station in Pacific Grove, the University of Chicago, and the Institute for Molecular Biophysiology of Florida State University in Tallahassee.

**Mercedes Gaffron** (born July 2, 1908, Lima, Peru; died February 19, 1993, Durham, NC), an art historian and good friend of Hanna Ruestow. She received her PhD from the University of Berlin in 1934, and her MD in 1939 from the University of Munich. She moved from Munich to Durham in 1948.

**Stefan George** (born July 12, 1868, Bingen, Germany; died December 4, 1933, Locarno, Switzerland), a poet and writer whose works were an important bridge between the nineteenth century and German modernism.

**Edit Ullstein Glaser** (born March 11, 1905, Berlin; died December 29, 1964, Durham, NC), the daughter of Hermann Ullstein, youngest of five brothers who owned the Ullstein Verlag, a large and prestigious publishing company in Berlin. Documents concerning the Ullstein family are contained chiefly in the Axel-Springer Verlag in Berlin; others are in the Stefan George Archiv, Württembergische Landesbibliothek in Stuttgart.

**Ernst Gundolf** (born December 24, 1881, Darmstadt; died May 15, 1945, London), the younger brother of Friedrich Gundolf, was an artist and member of George's circle. Although he himself published little, he was an astute critical reader whose opinions were valued by this group.

**Friedrich Gundolf** (born June 20, 1880, Darmstadt; died July 12, 1931, Heidelberg), a literary historian famous for his work on Caesar, Goethe, Shakespeare, and George, and George's closest companion for many years. He taught for much of his career at the University of Heidelberg.

**Frederic Hanes** (born September 18, 1883, Winston-Salem, NC; died March 25, 1946, Winston-Salem, NC), a member of a North Carolina family whose fortune came from tobacco and textiles. He was a physician and chairman of the Department of Medicine at Duke from 1933 until his death in 1946.

**Elizabeth Gilmore Holt** (born July 5, 1905, San Francisco; died January 25, 1987, Washington, DC), studied art history at the Universities of Wisconsin and Harvard, and continued her studies in Florence, Berlin, and Munich, where she received her PhD in 1934. She was editor of the Documentary History of Art series.

**Julian Huxley** (born June 22, 1887, London; died February 14, 1975, London), the brother of Aldous Huxley and grandson of Thomas H. Huxley, was a biologist, writer, and philosopher.

**Martin Jacoby** (born 1872, Berlin; died 1941, London), director, from 1906 to 1934, of the chemical institute of the Moabit Hospital in Berlin.

**Ernst Kantorowicz** (born May 3, 1895, Posen; died September 9, 1963, Princeton), a member of George's circle, taught medieval history at the University of Frankfurt am Main. After leaving Germany in 1938 he joined the faculty at the University of California, Berkeley. He left Berkeley over the Loyalty Oath controversy and spent the rest of his academic career at the Institute for Advanced Study in Princeton.

**Angelika Munk Kempner** (born 1835, Glogau, Germany; died 1915, Berlin), Walter Kempner's paternal grandmother, was a woman of considerable musical talent and a fine singing voice. She was known in Glogau as the "Silesian Nightingale."

**Benedicta Kempner** (born July 8, 1904, Steige, Germany; died May 4, 1982, Frankfurt am Main), the wife of Robert Kempner. Born Ruth Hahn, she converted to Catholicism after her marriage and took the name Benedicta Maria Kempner. Under this name she wrote two books on the nuns and priests of Germany under the Hitler regime.

**Lydia Rabinowitsch Kempner** (born August 22, 1871, Kovno [then Poland, now Lithuania]; died August 3, 1935, Berlin), the mother of Walter, Robert, and Nadja Kempner.

**Nadja Kempner** (born April 25, 1901, Berlin; died October 3, 1932, Berlin), received her PhD from the University of Heidelberg.

**Robert Kempner** (born October 9, 1899, Freiburg; died August 15, 1993, Frankfurt am Main).

**Walter Kempner, Sr.** (born June 17, 1864, Glogau, Germany; died March 1, 1920, Berlin), father of Walter, Robert, and Nadja Kempner. From a prominent Jewish family in Glogau. He graduated from medical school at the University of Berlin and worked as a physician without pay at the Institut für Hygiene in Munich and the Senckenberg Institute of the Goethe University in Frankfurt am Main before joining the Koch Institute in 1896.

**Ancel Keys** (born January 26, 1904, Colorado Springs; died November 20, 2004, Minneapolis), earned a PhD in oceanography and biology and a second PhD in physiology at Cambridge University. He was closely associated with two famous diets: balanced meals for combat soldiers in World War II (named "K-rations" after him) and the Mediterranean diet.

**Robert Koch** (born December 11, 1843, Clausthal, Germany; died May 27, 1910, Baden-Baden), earned his medical degree at the University of Göttingen, then worked with Rudolf Virchow in Berlin. A founder of the science of bacteriology and a major pioneer in the field of infectious diseases, he established the tubercle bacillus as the cause of tuberculosis. He was recipient of many medals, honorary doctorates, and prizes, including the 1905 Nobel Prize for Physiology.

**Willem Kolff** (born February 14, 1911, Leiden, Netherlands; died February 11, 2009, Newtown Square, PA), a Dutch physician, developed the dialysis machine during World War II in his efforts to treat Dutch soldiers suffering kidney failure. He first published reports on this work in 1944, and in 1947 he visited major medical centers in the United States to promote his new machine. He was later instrumental in the development of the artificial heart.

**Käthe Kollwitz** (born July 8, 1867, Königsberg, East Prussia [now Russia]; died April 22, 1945, Moritzburg), an artist best known for her drawings, particularly in charcoal, many of which were intimate portraits of people suffering in war. She and her husband, Karl, a prominent physician, lost two sons in World War I.

**Friedrich Krauss** (born September 29, 1900, Riga, Latvia; died June 24, 1977, Munich), received his PhD in the history of architecture. He was a professor at Munich's Technische Hochschule and published on the ancient sites of Paestum and Miletus. He met Mercedes Gaffron in Paestum in the 1930s, when she was studying art, and for over 40 years shared a house in Munich with her and Hanna Ruestow.

**Ludolf Krehl** (born December 26, 1861, Leipzig; died May 26, 1937, Heidelberg), director of the medical clinic of the University of Heidelberg when Walter Kempner studied there.

**Mary Lasker** (born November 30, 1900, Watertown, WI; died February 21, 1994, Greenwich, CT), a powerful philanthropist and citizen lobbyist who advocated for increased funding for medical research. She was also renowned for her work in urban beautification. She and her husband Albert Lasker created the Lasker Foundation in 1942 for the support of medical research and health programs.

**Ruth Lohmann Peschel** (born December 28, 1904, Berlin; died December 28, 1986, Durham, NC).

**Helen Mertens** (born September 24, 1910, Berlin; died December 30, 1997, Durham, NC).

**George Minot** (born December 2, 1885, Boston; died February 25, 1950, Brookline, MA), a professor of medicine at Harvard University, specializing in hematology. He received the 1934 Nobel Prize for Medicine for his treatment of pernicious anemia.

**Otto Morgenstern** (born February 2, 1860, Magdeburg, Germany; died November 28, 1942, Theresienstadt, Germany [now Czech Republic]), a teacher in the Schiller gymnasium who taught both Robert and Walter Kempner. He was in a group rounded up by the Nazis and deported to a concentration camp, where he was killed. After the war, a street in the west Berlin suburb of Steglitz-Zehlendorf was named in his honor.

**Ernst Morwitz** (born September 13, 1887, Danzig; died September 20, 1971, Minusio, Locarno), a poet and one of Stefan George's circle of scholars, was a judge in the Prussian Supreme Court.

**Katherine Ormston** (born January 6, 1908, Pittsburgh; died August 22, 1995, Durham, NC), a patient on the rice diet who became a member of Dr. Kempner's staff.

**Johannes Orth** (born January 14, 1847, Wallmerod, Germany; died January 13, 1923, Berlin), a physician and Rudolf Virchow's successor as head of the Institute of Pathology at the Charité Hospital in Berlin. A specialist in infectious diseases, particularly tuberculosis, he defended Lydia Rabinowitsch's findings that bovine tuberculosis was pathogenic in humans.

**Olga Marx Perlzweig** (born February 15, 1894, New York; died October 21, 1988, New York), the wife of William Perlzweig and mother of Judith Perlzweig Binder.

**William A. Perlzweig** (born April 23, 1891, Ostrog, Russia; died December 10, 1949, Durham, NC), a biochemist interested in nutrition. He taught at Columbia, the Rockefeller Institute, and Johns Hopkins before becoming a member of the founding faculty of Duke University Medical School.

**Ernst Peschel** (born December 5, 1902, Dessau; died January 2, 1987, Durham, NC).

**Gerda von Puttkamer** (born February 1901, Karzin, Pomerania; died November 27, 1953, Freiburg im Breisgau), nicknamed "Puma" by Friedrich Gundolf because with a simple twist her name became *Pumkater*, or puma cat. In 1927 she married Karl Schlayer, brother of Clotilde Schlayer.

**Christa Zielke von Roebel** (born April 22, 1904, Stolp; died May 14, 1968, Durham, NC), studied medicine in Heidelberg and after the war directed the obstetrics and gynecology clinic in Leipzig.

**Horst von Roebel** (born January 11, 1896, Königsberg; died December 12, 1964, Bad Godesberg), the husband of Christa Zielke, head of the Forberg music publishing firm in Leipzig (later relocated to Bonn).

**Fides Ruestow** (born May 30, 1910, Leipzig; died October 28, 2004, Durham, NC), sister of Hanna Ruestow.

**Hanna Ruestow** (born June 14, 1916, Munich; died June 28, 2002, Durham, NC).

**Alexander Schlayer** (born March 23, 1929, Freiburg), the son of Gerda and Karl Schlayer. In 1962 he settled in Sweden, where he taught languages in a high school for over 30 years.

**Clotilde Schlayer** (born December 18, 1900, Barcelona; died November 18, 2004, Durham, NC).

**Felix Schlayer** (born November 20, 1873, Reutlingen; died November 25, 1950, Madrid), husband of Roas Albagés y Gallego and father of Clotilde and Karl Schlayer.

**Karl Schlayer** (born December 18, 1900, Barcelona; died November 17, 1987, Madrid), Clotilde Schlayer's twin brother, was a physicist.

**Barbara Zielke Schultz** (born May 20, 1901, Stolp; died October 26, 1988, Durham, NC), sister of Christa Zielke von Roebel and wife of Hans Stefan Schultz.

**Hans Stefan Schultz** (born February 12, 1905, Halle; died November 19, 1984, Durham, NC), a classical philologist, received his undergraduate degree from Williams College as an exchange student and his PhD (1931) from the University of Berlin. He was a relative of the Henkell champagne family and also of von Ribbentrop.

**Helen Starke** (born January 2, 1918, Bronx, NY; died July 11, 1995, Maryknoll, NY).

**Claus von Stauffenberg** (born November 15, 1907, Jettingen, Swabia; died July 20, 1944, Berlin), a member of the German nobility and a career military officer. He met George in 1923 and became a member of his circle. After his participation in a failed attempt to assassinate Hitler, he was executed in the courtyard of the Bendlerblock, Berlin's Nazi headquarters.

**Eugene A. Stead, Jr.** (born October 6, 1908, Atlanta; died June 12, 2005, Bullock, NC), best known as a medical educator, researcher, and the founder of the Physician Assistant program. He served on the medical faculty at Harvard, Emory (where he received a Bachelor of Science and MD degree), and Duke Universities. His research in the 1940s paved the way for cardiac catheterization in medicine.

**William Stern** (born April 29, 1871, Berlin; died March 27, 1938, Durham, NC), a psychologist noted for his development of the Intelligence Quotient (IQ test), was one of the endangered scholars rescued from the Nazis by the Rockefeller program. He was relocated to Duke University.

**Ludwig Thormaehlen** (born May 24, 1889, Hanau; died May 3, 1956, Bad Ems), an art historian and sculptor, was a member of George's circle. For a time he was director of the National Gallery in Berlin, but was fired in the purge of "decadent" artists [who did not conform to the Nazis' nationalistic ideals].

**Charlotte Tilley** (born June 1, 1929, Durham, NC; died October 10, 1988, Durham, NC).

**Berthold Vallentin** (born February 13, 1877, Berlin; died March 13, 1933, Berlin), a lawyer and scholar who wrote poetry and biography, was a member of Stefan George's circle. He was married to Walter Kempner's aunt, Diana Rabinowitsch, an actress with the stage name Fanny Ritter.

**Rudolf Ludwig Karl Virchow** (born October 13, 1821, Schivelbein, Pomerania; died September 5, 1902, Berlin), a prominent German physician as well as a distinguished anthropologist and ethnologist. He played a prominent role in establishing a modern health care system in Berlin.

**Franz Volhard** (born May 2, 1872, Munich; died May 24, 1950, Frankfurt am Main), studied medicine in Bonn, Strasbourg, and Halle. A leading clinician in the first half of the 20th century, he classified Bright's disease.

**Otto Warburg** (born October 8, 1863, Freiburg; died August 1, 1970, West Berlin).

**Ernst von Weizsäcker** (born May 25, 1882, Stuttgart; died August 4, 1951, Lindau), a German diplomat from 1920–38 and secretary of state from 1938–43. He was a reluctant collaborator with the Nazis.

**Paul Dudley White** (born June 6, 1886, Roxbury, Massachusetts; died October 31, 1973, Boston), a cardiologist who stressed prevention through healthy living and exercise. He received his undergraduate and medical education at Harvard University. He is best known to the public as the physician who treated President Eisenhower's cardiac infarct.

**Karl Wolfskehl** (born September 17, 1869, Darmstadt; died June 30, 1948, Auckland, New Zealand), a poet and writer in Munich, was a member of George's circle. He emigrated in 1933 to Italy, and thence to New Zealand in 1938, where he lived the rest of his life. His gravestone in the Jewish cemetery in Auckland bears the inscription "exul poeta," exiled poet.

**Karl Zener** (born April 22, 1903, Indianapolis; died September 27, 1964, Durham, NC), an American psychologist who studied at Harvard and Princeton Universities and later, on a National Research Council Fellowship, at the University of Berlin. He joined the Duke Department of Psychology in 1928 and was its chairman from 1961 to 1964. His interest was in the biological aspect of psychology, with a special interest in perception.

# Glossary

**Acid-base balance.** The ratio of acid to alkali (base) in body fluids; maintenance of a healthy ratio is necessary for healthy function.

**Amino acids.** The building blocks of proteins.

**Aneurysm.** A permanent dilation or bulge in the wall of the heart or blood vessel due to a weakening of the wall and/or pressure on the wall.

**Anoxemia.** Absence of oxygen.

**Ascites.** Accumulation of fluids in the abdominal cavity.

**Bacillus.** A rod-shaped microorganism (bacterium).

**Bacillus abortus.** A bacterium that causes abortion in cattle.

**Cantharidin.** A chemical substance used to produce inflammatory blisters.

**Deamination.** Removal of a nitrogen (amine) group; deamination occurs during the breakdown of amino acids.

**Electrolyte.** Any substance that dissociates into ions in solution and therefore conducts electricity, e.g., sodium chloride, potassium chloride.

**Enzymes.** Proteins that facilitate or accelerate chemical reactions.

**Erythroblasts.** Primitive red blood cells.

**Exudates.** Fluids, especially inflammatory fluids, accumulating outside the blood vessels.

**Eyeground.** The interior of the eyeball, where blood vessels and the optic nerve are visible and can be photographed.

**Fermentation.** The chemical reaction by which living cells break down organic compounds to simple substances, e.g., carbon dioxide and alcohol.

**Glycolysis.** The breakdown of sugars to produce energy.

**Hematology.** The scientific study of blood.

**Inflammation.** Reaction of body tissue to injury, grossly expressed as swelling and redness.

**Lactic acid.** Product formed during glycolysis.

**Leukemia.** Disease characterized by excess of immature white blood cells.

**Manometer.** An instrument for measuring pressure of gases and liquids.

**Metabolism.** The breakdown and synthesis of substances necessary to sustain living organisms.

**Myeloblasts.** Primitive white blood cells.

**Nephritis.** Acute or chronic kidney inflammation, usually marked by high blood pressure and red blood cells in the urine; may cause uremia (*q.v.*).

**Nephrosis.** Kidney disease characterized by swelling, high cholesterol and low protein in serum, and excess protein in urine. Blood pressure is usually unaffected.

**Oxygen tension.** Oxygen concentration or pressure.

**Pathogenic.** Causing disease.

**Phlorhizin.** A glucoside compound, derived from root bark of fruit trees, that can be used to produce a type of diabetes in animals.

**Plasma.** The cell-free component of blood.

**PSP (phenolsulfonphthalein).** Chemical introduced by injection into the blood stream and excreted in the urine; used to measure kidney function.

**Renal.** Pertaining to the kidney.

**Respiration.** The chemical process by which nutrients are oxidized and broken down to carbon dioxide and water with a net gain of energy.

**Sympathectomy.** Surgical removal of the sympathetic ganglia (collections of nerve cell bodies along the spinal cord) in order to increase blood flow.

**Uremia.** Toxic accumulation of nitrogenous waste products in the blood stream occurring in renal failure.

# Index

Note: *f* denotes figure; *n* denotes footnote.